BODY FLUIDS
AND ELECTROLYTES

A PROGRAMMED PRESENTATION

BODY FLUIDS AND ELECTROLYTES

A PROGRAMMED PRESENTATION

NORMA JEAN WELDY, R.N., B.S., M.S.

Professor of Nursing, Goshen College
Goshen, Indiana

SIXTH EDITION

with 35 illustrations and 6 tables

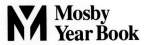
Mosby
Year Book

St. Louis Baltimore Boston Chicago London Philadelphia Sydney Toronto

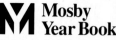
Mosby
Year Book
Dedicated to Publishing Excellence

Executive Editor: Don Ladig
Developmental Editor: Robin Carter
Project Manager: Carol Sullivan Wiseman
Production Editor: Lisa D. Cohen
Book and Cover Design: Gail Morey Hudson
Cover Illustrator: Mark Swindle

SIXTH EDITION

Previous editons copyrighted 1972, 1976, 1980, 1984, 1988

Printed in the United States of America

Mosby–Year Book, Inc., 11830 Westline Industrial Drive, St. Louis, Missouri 63146

Library of Congress Cataloging in Publication Data

Weldy, Norma Jean.
    Body fluids and electrolytes : a programmed presentation / Norma Jean Weldy. — 6th ed.
      p.   cm.
    Includes bibliographical references and index.
    ISBN 0-8016-5577-3
    1. Body fluid disorders—Nursing—Programmed instruction.
    2. Water-electrolyte imbalances—Nursing—Programmed instruction.
    3. Water-electrolyte balance (Physiology)—Programmed instruction.
    I. Title.
RC630.W45   1992
612′.01522′077—dc20   91-22162
                                       CIP

CL/DC 9 8 7 6 5 4 3

Preface

This text is designed to assist nursing students in overcoming some of the confusion about body fluids and electrolytes. A comprehension of body fluids and electrolytes is essential to understanding many clinical conditions. Nursing students who have a better knowledge of body fluids and electrolytes will give more holistic nursing care to patients. This text is designed for students in nursing who have some basic theoretical knowledge of the biological sciences from their high school curriculum. Students who have had further study of anatomy, physiology, and chemistry will be able to proceed more rapidly through the program. The percentages and laboratory values relate to infants, children, young and middle-aged adults, and elderly persons.

The information is given in sequence, from simple to complex. Each step builds on previous learning. There are written summaries followed by review questions throughout the book. These are presented to help the learner decide when to move on to the next section.

Programmed material does not replace the need for a live teacher, but it does present organized information that students can use to learn at their own rate. The teacher will have to decide how to use this program most effectively. I have found classroom discussion useful after the students have completed the program; I then assign them to care for patients. That is followed by seminar discussion in which they discuss case presentations involving various types of fluid and electrolyte imbalance, the signs and symptoms observed, and the nursing care indicated.

The ultimate objective of the program is to develop in nursing students the ability:

1. To use basic technical terms
2. To recognize the need for an accurate clinical estimate of fluid balance
   a. To measure and record fluid intake and output when indicated
   b. To weigh the patient daily when indicated
3. To identify patients likely to have fluid and electrolyte imbalance and to recognize and report the signs and symptoms
4. To identify patients likely to retain sodium and to recognize and report the signs and symptoms
5. To identify patients likely to lose potassium and to recognize and report the signs and symptoms
6. To recognize and report the signs and symptoms of dehydration
7. To identify patients likely to develop a magnesium imbalance and to recognize and report the signs and symptoms
8. To identify patients likely to develop a calcium imbalance and to recognize and report the signs and symptoms
9. To institute nursing measures to minimize imbalance
   a. To replace fluids and electrolytes
      (1) To encourage and provide oral intake in specific amounts
      (2) To know shy fluids are essential
      (3) To measure and record intake and output when indicated
      (4) To provide additional fluid before placing the patient on an order of "nothing by mouth"
      (5) To know how and when to force fluids
      (6) To regulate the flow of parenteral fluids safely

  b. To minimize loss of fluids and electrolytes
   (1) To observe and report loss
   (2) To limit the frequency of irrigations with a nasogastic tube and normal saline solutions
  c. To give medications intelligently

  I am especially pleased with the reception of the previous editions and would like to express my appreciation to the many persons who have helped to make the present edition possible. Your questions, comments, and suggestions have been incorporated in this edition. I have discovered that the book is being used as a reference as well as a classroom text. Therefore an index has been included.

  In this sixth edition I have changed some of the terminology to reflect the use of the nursing process. References to assessment data that can be obtained and suggested nursing diagnoses have been added. Most of the cases included do not contain enough specific information about any individual to be able to formulate a nursing diagnosis. A nursing diagnosis is focused on the diagnosis and treatment of the client's responses that the nurse can treat legally and independently. Many of the physiological needs of a person with either fluid and/or electrolyte imbalance require orders by a physician and are therefore collaborative or interdependent problems. For collaborative or interdependent problems, nurses assess, monitor, detect, and report their observations and assessment. Two tables have been added, as well as a summary of assessment data.

Norma Jean Weldy

Norma Jean Weldy

To the student

This is a program to help you understand the need for balance in body fluids and electrolytes. It will help you learn terms necessary in understanding fluid and electrolyte balance. It will help you understand where fluids and electrolytes are located in the body and how they move. You should gain information on how fluids and electrolytes are lost and how they are replaced both in health and in disease. Through this study, you should learn to recognize the signs and symptoms that indicate imbalance of fluids or electrolytes.

The program will help you learn about some of the laboratory tests that indicate imbalance and some common methods of treating the imbalance. Also, you should learn what is important in giving nursing care to patients who have, or may have, an imbalance in fluids or electrolytes.

Each statement or paragraph is called a frame. At the end of each frame, there is a question with a place for you to respond. The answers are given in the left-hand column. As you work through the program, read carefully and completely formulate your answers to the questions before you look at the answer given. Use the template provided to cover the answer column. If you have questions, consult your instructor.

There are four types of statements to be completed:

1. Sometimes there is a blank to complete the statement. If so, write your answer in the blank and

then compare it with the correct response in the answer column.

2. Sometimes you will need to make a choice from two or three answers. Those statements are written as follows:

This book (will? will not?) help you understand body fluids and electrolytes. Circle the correct choice and compare your response with the answer column.

3. Some statements ask you to respond to questions or situations in your own words. Check your written answer with the suggestions made in the answer column. Your answer does not have to be identical, but it must contain the same idea.

4. Some statements ask you to select the right answers from a list of several possible answers. Make a check by the correct answers and compare your response with the answer column.

Contents

BODY FLUIDS
AND ELECTROLYTES

A PROGRAMMED PRESENTATION

PART 1

Fluid and electrolyte balance

INTRODUCTION

People cannot live without body fluid. Water is the largest single constituent of the body. In the average young to middle-aged adult the total body fluid amounts to about 60% of the body weight, and in a newborn infant, 70% to 75% of the total body weight is fluid. By the age of 2 years, the percent of body weight that is fluid is approximately the same as that of a young to middle-aged adult, 60%. In the elderly, because of changes in body tissues, the total body fluid drops to 45% to 50% of body weight. Because of the high percentage of body weight that is fluid, in infants, fluid balance is extremely important. Since the elderly have a much lower percentage of body weight that is fluid, they are also highly likely to develop fluid imbalance. One of the important functions of the nurse is to assess the patient's fluid balance or imbalance. When a person vomits, he loses some of the normal fluid content of the body. If the vomiting continues and he does not drink fluids, the loss may become serious. The person becomes lethargic, the mucous membranes become dry, and the body temperature increases. A person becomes very uncomfortable when the body's fluid content is less than normal.

A loss of 20% of the fluid content is *fatal*. For example, a person with third-degree burns over a major area of the body will lose fluid through seepage from the burned areas. If the fluid is not replaced, he will die. By replacing the body fluid, the nurse can make the person more comfortable and may save his life.

1 From a study of anatomy and physiology we know that body fluids have two main functions. One of the functions of body fluids is to provide transportation of nutrients to the cells and carry waste products from the cells.

transportation of nutrients
and waste products

One function of body fluids is _____

_____.

2 A second major function of body fluids is to provide a medium in which chemical reactions can occur.

Body fluids provide for transport of nutrients and waste products, and they are also necessary so that

chemical reactions

_____ can occur.

BODY FLUID COMPARTMENTS

3 Body fluids are contained within three compartments. These compartments are not bladders tucked away somewhere, but the term *compartment* is a convenient abstraction used to describe where fluid is found in the body. Most of the body fluids are inside the cells, and we call this the intracellular compartment. *Intra-* is a prefix meaning within, or on the inside. When we give intramuscular injections, we give the medication within, or inside, the muscle.

The largest amount of body fluids is within the cell

intracellular

and is called _____.

4 The fluid in each cell has its own unique composition, but the concentration of intracellular constituents is similar from one cell to another cell. If you have three kinds of cookies, each cookie may contain different ingredients; but even though they are not alike in composition, we call each of them a cookie, or three cookies. Although the intracellular fluid of individual cells differs in chemical composition, it is similar in concentration. Therefore the intracellular fluid of all the different cells may be considered one large fluid compartment, even though it is contained in individual cells.

a The concentration of constituents in each cell is (the

similar

same? similar? different?).

composition

b Each cell has its own chemical _____.

5 We may use the term *extracellular* to refer to all the fluid outside the cells. The prefix *extra-* means outside of. In school we participate in extracurricular activities. Extracurricular activities are those pursuits that are not a part of the student's course of study but are important for learning. Extracellular means outside the cell.

intracellular   **a** Fluid that is *within* the cell is called _____.

extracellular   **b** Fluid that is *outside* the cell is called _____.

6 The *extracellular* fluid is outside the cell, but part of that fluid is within the blood vessels.

Since *intra-* means within and *-vascular* means vessel, the fluid that is within blood vessels is called

intravascular   _____.

7 Although some of the extracellular fluid is within the blood vessels (intravascular), the rest of the extracellular fluid is between the cells. Since this fluid is *between* the cells and blood vessels, it is called *interstitial* fluid.

Therefore the extracellular fluid is divided into two parts:

intravascular   **a** (within blood vessels) _____

interstitial   **b** (between cells) _____

8 If we divide all body fluid into only two groups, we use the cell as our point of reference; so fluids are either inside the cell or outside the cell.

The two main compartments for body fluids are

intracellular   **a** (inside the cell) _____

extracellular   **b** (outside the cell) _____

9 We can then divide the extracellular fluids into two groups, those within the blood vessels and those between the cells.

intravascular   The former group is called _____,

interstitial   and the latter _____.

10 The fluid compartments are separated by semipermeable membranes. Since the fluids outside the cells (intravascular and interstitial) are constantly mixing through the capillary walls, the extracellular fluid is contained within a communicating chamber.

mixing   The extracellular fluids are (mixing? separate?).

11 Label the body fluid compartments in the blanks at the left of the diagram.

Extracellular
Intracellular
Interstitial
Intravascular

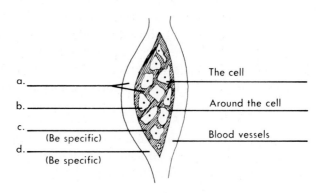

a. _____

b. _____

c. _____
(Be specific)

d. _____
(Be specific)

The cell

Around the cell

Blood vessels

DISTRIBUTION OF BODY FLUIDS

12 Study the figure below and answer the following questions:

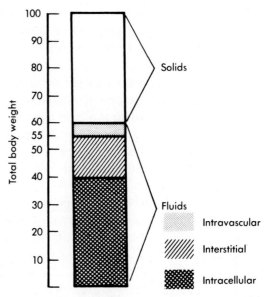

% Body weight in children and young to middle-aged adults

60%

40

a The percent of total body weight that is fluid is ____.

b The fluid inside the cells is ____% of body weight.

5

c The fluid within the blood vessels is _____% of body weight.

13 Newborn infants have a higher proportion of body weight that is fluid than do children and adults. Up to age 2 years, the proportion of body weight that is fluid is from 70% to 75%.

70% to 75%

In infants the percent of total body weight that is fluid is _____.

14 In infants the percent of fluid inside the cell is 40% of body weight, the same as in young to middle-aged adults. In infants the extracellular fluid is approximately 35% of body weight.

35%

The percent of total body weight that is extracellular fluid in infants is approximately _____.

15 With age, the total body water diminishes. In the elderly the intracellular fluid is reduced because of tissue loss. The percent of total body weight that is fluid may be reduced to 45% to 50% in persons over age 65.

45%

A person aged 65 is likely to have (45%? 60%? 75%?) of body weight that is fluid.

16 The body must have fluid to continue its normal processes. The kidneys excrete the largest quantity of fluid, but fluid also leaves the body through the gastrointestinal tract, lungs and skin.

kidneys

Fluid normally leaves the body through the gastrointestinal tract, lungs, skin, and _____.

17 The fluid in the body is replenished in two ways. The most obvious is by the ingestion of liquids; but, in addition, meats and vegetables contain 60% to 97% water. Also, the breakdown of food yields water of oxidation. (Water is one of the products of metabolism.) About 10 ml of water is released by the metabolism of each 100 calories of fat, carbohydrate, or protein.

metabolism (water of oxidation)

Two sources of fluid for the body are ingestion of liquids and the water in foods. The third source of fluids is by _____.

CONSTITUENTS OF BODY FLUIDS

Electrolytes

18 The body fluids consist of water and dissolved substances. Some substances such as glucose, urea, and creatinine do not dissociate in solution. That is, they do not separate from their complex form into simpler substances when they are in a solution.

does not   Glucose (does? does not?) dissociate when in solution.

19 Although some substances do not dissociate when in solution, other substances do dissociate. For example, when sodium chloride (NaCl) is in a solution, it dissociates, or separates, into two parts or elements.

Some   (Some? All?) substances dissociate when in solution.

20 Before further discussion of body fluid constituents, we shall consider some of the terms being used. Remember: an *atom* is the smallest particle of an element that still has the properties of the element. When two or more atoms combine to form a substance, this is called a *molecule*. Atoms are composed of particles. The particles of an atom are the *proton*, *neutron*, and *electron*. The proton carries a positive charge, the electron carries a negative charge of the same magnitude, and the neutron is neutral.[11] You can remember that the neutron is neutral because "neutron" and "neutral" begin with the same five letters. You can remember that the proton carries a positive charge because both "proton" and "positive" begin with the letter "p." That leaves only the electron to remember as being different.

negative   **a** The electron of an atom carries a (positive? negative? neutral?) charge.

positive   **b** The proton of an atom carries a (positive? negative? neutral?) charge.

21 The proton and neutron are in the nucleus, or center, of the atom.

    Therefore the nucleus is positively charged because it contains both the neutron, which is neutral, and the

proton   (proton? electron?), which is positive.

22 Electrons carry negative charges and revolve around

the nucleus. As long as the number of electrons in an atom is the same as the number of protons, there is no net charge on the atom (i.e., it is neither positive nor negative). However, atoms may gain, lose, or share electrons and then no longer be neutral.

If an atom either gains or loses electrons, it is no longer _____.

neutral

23 When an atom carries an electrical charge because it has either gained or lost electrons, we call it an *ion*. An ion is an electrically charged atom or group of atoms.

An atom that has an electrical charge is called a/an _____.

ion

24 An ion may carry either a positive or a negative charge. When an ion carries a positive charge, it is called a *cation*.

A cation is an ion with a (positive? negative?) electrical charge.

positive

25 Another way to explain an ion with a positive charge, or a cation, is that this ion is an electron donor. It has given away, or lost, electrons. The result is fewer electrons than protons. Since the protons carry the positive charge and the electrons the negative charge, and this ion has given away electrons, the result is a positive charge.

A cation carries a positive electrical charge because it has given away _____.

electrons

26 It may help you to remember that cations are positive ions if you see that "cation" has a "t" (or +) in it. A cation is an ion that carries a positive electrical charge. However, not all ions are cations. Some ions carry a negative electrical charge. When an ion has gained, or taken on, electrons, it assumes a negative charge. Since the electrons are negatively charged, and we have now added electrons, the result is a negatively charged ion.

Negatively charged ions have (gained? lost?) electrons.

gained

27 An ion that has gained electrons and therefore carries a negative charge is called an anion.

negative

positive

a Anions carry _____ electrical charges.

b A cation carries a _____ electrical charge.

28 Another term we shall use is *electrolyte*. When a substance is dissolved in solution and some of its molecules split or dissociate into electrically charged atoms, or ions, we call that substance an electrolyte. If we take an electrolyte such as sodium chloride (NaCl) and dissolve it in solution, it will dissociate into sodium (Na^+) and chloride (Cl^-).

Sodium is the cation because it carries a positive charge. Chloride carries a negative charge and is called

anion

the _____.

29 Electrolytes are the substances we have been discussing that dissociate in solution into electrically

ions

charged atoms called _____.

30 An electrolyte dissociates into electrically charged ions when in solution. Therefore, when an electrolyte is dissolved in water, it conducts an electrical current. We can demonstrate this by placing two electrodes in an electrolyte solution and connecting them to a bulb and battery. The dissociation of the electrolyte into charged atoms or ions will conduct an electrical current between the electrodes. The anion, the negatively charged ion, will migrate to the anode, which is the electrode with a positive charge. Remember: positive charges attract negative charges, whereas like charges repel. Therefore the negative ion (anion) will be attracted to the anode.

positive

The anion ($-$) will be attracted to the (positive? negative?) electrode.

31 The positive electrode is called the *anode*, and anions ($-$) will migrate to it. The negative electrode is called the *cathode*, and cations ($+$) will be attracted to it.

positive

The cation is the (positive? negative?) ion.

32 The cation is the positive ion and will be attracted to the cathode.

negative

Therefore the cathode is the (positive? negative?) electrode.

33 Those ions that carry a positive charge are called *cations* (+) and are attracted to the cathode (−) when electricity passes through a solution. The ions carrying a negative charge are called *anions* (−) and are attracted to the anode (+).

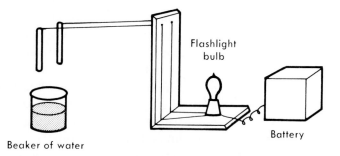

Flashlight bulb

Battery

Beaker of water

If we put sodium chloride (NaCl) in a beaker and raise the beaker so the electrodes are immersed in the solution,

a What will happen to demonstrate that electricity has been conducted?_____

The bulb will light.

_____

cathode

b Where will the sodium (Na^+) go? To the (cathode? anode?).

anode

c Where will the chloride (Cl^-) go? To the (cathode? anode?).

Measurement of electrolytes

34 To study body fluids, we must have suitable units of measurement. To measure volume of fluids, we use the metric system and measure in liters (L) or milliliters (ml). A milliliter is one thousandth of a liter and is generally considered the same as a cubic centimeter (cc). Therefore we may say that a liter is equal to 1000 cc. In common usage 1 cc is equal to 1 ml.

¹⁄₁₀₀₀

A milliliter is what fraction of a liter? (¹⁄₁₀? ¹⁄₁₀₀? ¹⁄₁₀₀₀?).

35 We must have a unit of measure for the various electrolytes in the body fluid. Since we are interested in the action of electrolytes (their ability to combine and form other compounds), the unit of measure must express

9

their combining power (chemical activity). The combining power is a function of the number of ions. The weight of the ion has no relation to the chemical activity of the ion. Measuring electrolytes in units of weight such as milligrams per 100 ml does not tell us the chemical combining power of the electrolytes in solution (i.e., how many cations, or positive ions, will be available to combine with anions, or negative ions). For example, if a hostess is having a party and wants couples of boys and girls, she does not invite 1000 pounds of boys for every 1000 pounds of girls. Their weight is not as important as the number of boys that will pair up with an equal number of girls. In measuring electrolytes, we are not concerned with how much they weigh (mg/100 ml). We want to know how many ions are available for chemical interaction. (An equal number of cations and anions is necessary.)

activity (combining power)

a We want to know the chemical _____ of the electrolytes in solution.

ions

b The chemical combining power of an electrolyte tells us how many _____ are available.

36 The unit of measure that expresses the combining activity of an electrolyte is the milliequivalent (mEq). An equivalent weight is the amount of one electrolyte that will displace or otherwise react with a given amount of hydrogen. Hydrogen is used as the yardstick or measure. One milliequivalent of any cation will always react chemically with 1 mEq of an anion, just as one boy reacts with one girl to make a couple.

100

a 100 mEq of cation will react chemically with _____ mEq of anion.

20

b 20 mEq of sodium (Na^+) will react with _____ mEq of chloride (Cl^-).

155

c If extracellular fluid has 155 mEq of cation, the number of milliequivalents of anion necessary for balance will be _____.

37 Milliequivalents provide information about the number of anions or cations available to combine with other cations or anions. For example, if the level of sodium cations in the blood is 140 mEq/L, this means that 140 cations are available to combine with 140 anions for each liter of blood. The average level of chloride ions in the blood is 104 mEq/L. Therefore, for each liter of blood, approximately 36 mEq of sodium is available to combine with some anion other than chloride.

The milliequivalent is a useful measure to compare

chemical activity
_____ of electrolytes.

38 The fluid in each of the compartments (intracellular, interstitial, and intravascular) contains electrolytes. Each compartment has a particular composition of electrolytes, which differs from that of the other compartments. To function normally, body cells must have fluids and electrolytes. Furthermore, the electrolytes must be in the right compartment in the right amount. If you put lettuce out in the sun, it will become wilted. You can make the lettuce crisp by placing it in salted ice water. In the body, when potassium is lost from the cell, the person becomes weak. If the potassium is not replaced, the person will die of myocardial necrosis and circulatory failure. (The heart muscle becomes soft, dies, and cannot pump blood, since the muscle and nerve fibers are not activated because of the lack of potassium within the cell.) A specific kind and amount of certain electrolytes must be available for normal cell function.

Normal function of body cells depends on the availability of certain _____.

electrolytes

39 When potassium is lost from the intracellular fluid, some other cation must replace it. Sodium, the most available cation in the extracellular fluid, moves into the cell.

equal (balanced)
a The anions and cations must be _____.

10
b 10 mEq of cations will react with exactly _____ mEq of anions.

SUMMARY

Fluids and electrolytes are essential for health. The fluid compartments are the intracellular and the extracellular; the extracellular compartment includes interstitial and intravascular fluids. The body fluids contain water and electrolytes, the substances that dissociate in water to electrically charged atoms called *ions*. The chemical combining power of an electrolyte is a measure of the number of ions. Electrolytes are measured in milliequivalents, which express their combining power. One milliequivalent of any cation will always react chemically with one 1 mEq of any anion. Whenever an electrolyte moves out of a cell, another electrolyte moves in to take its place. The number of cations and anions must be the same for homeostasis to exist.

REVIEW

1 The three fluid compartments in the body are

intracellular

a _____

intravascular

b _____

interstitial

c _____

substances that dissociate in solution into electrically charged particles called ions

2 Electrolytes are _____
_____
_____
_____.

chemical combining power

3 The number of ions available tells us the _____ _____ of an electrolyte.

the same number of

4 To achieve balance or equilibrium, we must have (more? the same number of? fewer?) anions than (as) cations.

Another cation moves in.

5 When one cation (e.g., K^+) moves out of a cell, what happens? _____
_____

NORMAL ELECTROLYTE COMPOSITION OF THE FLUID COMPARTMENTS

40 Refer to the diagrams on page 13 and answer the following questions:

a The major cation in both interstitial and intravascular

sodium

fluid is _____.

b The total milliequivalents of anion are equal to the

cation

milliequivalents of _____.

Electrolyte composition

Electrolyte composition of serum in intravascular compartment (mEq/L)

Electrolyte composition of interstitial fluid (mEq/L)

Electrolyte composition of intracellular fluid (mEq/L)

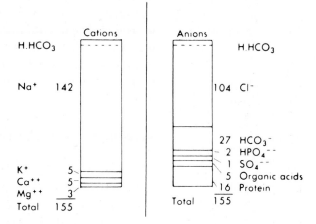

Intravascular

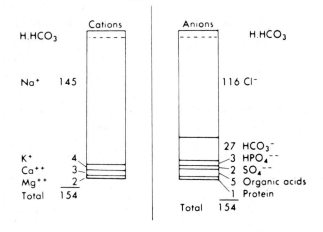

Interstitial

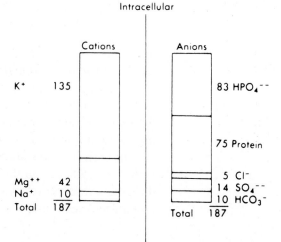

Intracellular

intracellular

potassium

less

chloride

c The fluid compartment that has the most protein is the _____.

d The chief cation in intracellular fluid is _____.

e There is (more? similar? less?) sodium in intracellular fluid than (as) in intravascular fluid.

f The chief anion in interstitial and intravascular fluid is _____.

MOVEMENT OF FLUID IN THE BODY

41 We have considered differences in composition of the intracellular, interstitial, and intravascular fluids. These differences in composition are partially due to the nature of the barriers that separate the fluids. Cell membranes separate the interstitial fluid from the intravascular fluid. However, these barriers are selectively permeable (i.e., the cell membrane and the capillary wall will allow water and some solutes free passage through them). The *solute* is the substance that is dissolved. For international travel you must have a passport to allow entrance into another country and return to your homeland; but certain countries, such as the United States and Canada, allow free passage without a passport. Accordingly, water and some solutes freely pass through the cell membrane and the capillary wall. We shall discuss later (frame 71) some ways in which the body requires a special transport system for certain substances.

unrestricted

Some

a Movement of water through the capillary wall is (unrestricted? restricted?).

b (Some? All?) solutes are allowed free passage through the walls of cells and capillaries.

42 There are several forces that affect the movement of water and solutes through the walls of cells and capillaries. We really have a mass-transportation system to carry the traffic between the fluid compartments. These forces must carry the molecules of water, foods, gases, wastes, and many kinds of ions. One process by which a solute (gas or substance) in solution moves is called *diffusion*. Diffusion is the movement of particles in all directions through a solution. When you pour a small amount of cream into a cup of black coffee, the cream mixes or spreads through the whole cup of coffee (i.e., diffuses throughout the coffee).

The process by which particles spread in all directions through a solution is called _____.

diffusion

43 Diffusion is the process by which a solute may spread throughout a solution or solvent. While a solute is the substance that is dissolved, a *solvent* is the solution in which the solute is dissolved.

solute

a A substance that is dissolved is called the (solute? solvent?).

b The solution in which a solute is dissolved is called the (solute? solvent?).

solvent

44 The particles (molecules or ions) of a substance dissolved in a solvent are moving continuously. If they are abundant in one area, they will bump into each other, causing the particles to spread from an area where there are more to an area where there are fewer particles. Thus molecules or ions diffuse from an area of high concentration to one of lower concentration.

Diffusion of a solute spreads the molecules from an area of high concentration to an area of _____ concentration.

lower

45 We have been discussing the diffusion of a solute throughout a solvent. Diffusion may also occur across a membrane if the membrane is permeable, or allows free passage. When a membrane is permeable to a certain substance, that substance can go through the membrane freely. A permeable membrane will allow substances to pass through it without restriction. However, all the membranes in the body are selectively permeable, or semipermeable.[1] A selectively permeable membrane will allow some solutes to pass through without restriction but will prevent other solutes from passing freely.

All the membranes in the body are (selectively? freely?) permeable to all substances.

selectively

46 Diffusion occurs within fluid compartments and from one compartment to another if the barrier between the compartments is permeable to the diffusing substances.

Diffusion is a very important process by which the solute and/or solvent may move freely from one fluid compartment to another. For example, the oxygen in the air we breathe enters the intravascular compartment and then the cells by diffusion.

some

One process for the movement of fluids and (some? all?) solutes is diffusion.

47 Now we shall consider another process, *osmosis*. If a membrane is permeable to water but not to all the solutes present, it is a selective or semipermeable membrane. When the solvent or water moves across this membrane, we call the process osmosis.

osmosis

The movement of fluid through a selectively permeable membrane is called _____.

48 Osmosis is the movement of solvent molecules across a membrane to an area where there is a higher concentration of solute that cannot pass through the membrane.

solvent

Osmosis is the movement of (solute? solvent?) across a selectively permeable membrane.

49

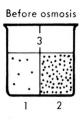

Before osmosis   After osmosis

1 = Dilute salt solution
2 = Concentrated salt solution
3 = Selectively permeable membrane

a Before osmosis the quantity of solution on both sides of the selectively permeable membrane is (different? the same?).

the same

b After osmosis the quantity of solution on both sides of the membrane is (different? equal?).

different

c (Solute? Solvent?) has moved.

Solvent

d The reason the solvent moved is that the membrane will not allow the solute to go through; therefore the membrane is (permeable? selectively permeable?).

selectively permeable

e After osmosis the concentration of salt solution on the two sides of the membrane is (the same? different?).

the same

50 All normal living membranes are selectively permeable (i.e., they do not allow all solutes free passage).

The movement of water through such membranes is

osmosis   by _____.

51 Earlier we established that particles move from an area of high concentration to an area of lower concentration. It may sound as though osmosis is the opposite. Remember, however, that a membrane is selective and allows the water to pass through but does not allow the solute through. So it is the water that is moving from an area where there is a greater amount of water in relation to solute to an area where there is less water in relation to solute.

The result of osmosis is two solutions, separated by a

equal   membrane, that are (equal? unequal?) in concentration.

52 When you have a more concentrated solution on one side of a selectively permeable membrane and a less concentrated solution on the other side, there is a pull called *osmotic pressure* that draws the water through the membrane to the more concentrated side, or the side with more solute.

Osmotic pressure is the force that draws the water from a less concentrated solution through a selectively

more   permeable membrane into a (less? equally? more?) concentrated solution.

53 The amount of osmotic pressure is determined by the relative number of particles of solute on the side of greater concentration. Therefore the greater the number of particles in the concentrated solution, the more pull there will be to move the water through the membrane.

The force that pulls water across the membrane from the side of a less concentrated solution into a more con-

osmotic pressure   centrated solution is called _____

_____.

54 When the solutions on both sides of a selectively permeable membrane have established equilibrium, or are equal in concentration, they are isotonic. *Iso-* is a combining form that means alike.

When the solutions on both sides of a selectively

permeable membrane are alike in concentration, they are

isotonic   _____.

55 One of the problems in clinical medicine is the maintenance of adequate body fluids and proper chemical balance between the intracellular and the extracellular fluids. The movement of water through the cell membrane normally occurs so rapidly that any lack of osmotic balance is corrected within seconds. Therefore a state of osmotic equilibrium is maintained constantly when the body is functioning normally. When an extracellular fluid has the same concentration as the intracellular fluid, there is no net shift of fluid from outside the cell to inside the cell. The term *net* means that which remains after the deduction of all loss or gain. There is some movement of fluid, but there is no resultant change in quantity.

isotonic   Therefore in this situation the extracellular fluid is like, or _____ with, the intracellular fluid.

56 An example of an isotonic solution is 0.85% sodium chloride, which is referred to as *isotonic saline* solution or *normal saline* solution. This means that it is isotonic to human cells and thus there will be very little osmosis.

0.85   An example of a solution that is isotonic to body cells is ____% sodium chloride.

57 Another example of an isotonic solution is 5% glucose.

will not be   When we say a solution is isotonic to another solution or to the intracellular fluid, we mean there (will be? will not be?) movement of fluid from one side of the membrane to the other side by osmosis.

58 When a solution contains a lower concentration of salt than another solution, we say it is hypotonic. *Hypo-* means less than ordinary. A hypotonic solution has less salt, or more water, than an isotonic solution.

less   A hypotonic solution has (more? less?) salt than an isotonic solution.

59 Distilled water is an example of a hypotonic solution, since it does not have solutes in it. If we put distilled water on one side of a selectively permeable membrane and normal saline solution (0.85% sodium chloride) on the other side, water will move from the distilled water side to the normal saline side to make the solutions on both sides of the membrane more nearly equal in concentration.

a hypotonic

Distilled water is an example of (a hypotonic? an isotonic?) solution.

60 We would never do this to a person, but if distilled water were injected into the bloodstream, the red blood cells would draw water into themselves. Since distilled water is hypotonic to the cells, osmosis would continue, in an attempt to bring about balance or equality, until the cells swelled and eventually burst if the situation were not changed.

swell

A cell placed in a very hypotonic solution will (swell? shrink?).

61 A solution that has a higher concentration of solutes than another solution is a hypertonic solution. We say a person who is overactive is hyperactive, *hyper-* meaning more than usual. A 10% solution of sodium chloride is an example of a hypertonic solution. A 10% solution of sodium chloride is too hypertonic to be injected into a person, but if we mix a 10% sodium chloride solution with red blood cells, water will move out of the cells and into the hypertonic solution. As the cells lose their fluid, they will become wrinkled and shriveled like prunes (i.e., crenated).

wrinkled and shriveled

Crenated means _____.

62 If either extreme (swelling or shriveling of the cells) occurs in a person, death will result. Fluids and electrolytes must be kept in balance for health. When they remain out of balance, death occurs. If a strong salt solution is injected into the extracellular fluid, water will be pulled out of the cells to go where the salt is.

a Shriveling happens because the salt solution is (hypotonic? hypertonic?) to the intracellular fluid.

hypertonic

hypotonic

b Swelling occurs if the cells are in a (hypotonic? hypertonic?) solution.

63 If the body loses more electrolytes than fluid, such as can happen in diarrhea, then the extracellular fluid will contain fewer electrolytes, or less solute, than the intracellular fluid.

pulled into
     Therefore the fluid will be (pulled into? pushed out of?) the cells.

64 The osmotic pressure of a solution is proportional to the number of particles per unit volume of solvent. The unit of measure of osmotic pressure is the *osmole*. Therefore the ability of solutes to cause osmosis and osmotic pressure is measured in terms of osmoles. In the body the osmole is too large a unit for satisfactory use in expressing osmotic activity. The term *milliosmole* (mosm), which equals ¹⁄₁₀₀₀ osmole, is used to measure osmotic pressure in the body.

milliosmoles
     In the body the osmotic pressure is measured in _____ (mosm).

65 *Osmolality* means the number of osmotically active particles per kilogram of water.

osmolality
     The osmotic pull of all particles per kilogram of water is called _____.

66 Osmolality refers to the number of osmotically active particles per kilogram of water. A closely related term, *osmolarity*, refers to the number of osmoles per liter solution.

osmolarity
     The osmotic pull of all particles per liter of solution is called _____.

67 In clinical practice the difference between osmolality and osmolarity is not significant. Osmolality is measured in milliosmoles per kilogram of water (mosm/kg) and osmolarity in milliosmoles per liter (mosm/L) This difference is negligible because of the low solute concentrations in body fluids.

is not
     The difference between osmolality and osmolarity (is? is not?) important in body fluids.

68 Another way to think about osmolality is as the "specific gravity" of body fluids. Since specific gravity is the weight of the solution compared with an equal volume of distilled water, the osmolality of a solution can be estimated by the specific gravity. However, the osmolality of urine is a more specific measure of renal function than the specific gravity. The kidneys respond to changes in osmolality rather than to changes in specific gravity. The normal osmolality of plasma is 280 to 294 mosm/kg.

280 to 294

The normal osmolality of plasma is _____ mosm/kg.

69 The osmolality of the extracellular fluid is determined mainly by the extracellular fluid concentration of sodium. Sodium is the most abundant extracellular cation and therefore provides 90% to 95% of the effective osmotic pressure of the extracellular fluid.

sodium

The osmolality of the extracellular fluid is determined mainly by _____.

70 Because of osmotic equilibrium, normally the extracellular fluid and the intracellular fluid have nearly the same osmolality.

280 to 294

Normal osmolality of plasma is _____ mosm/kg.

71 Diffusion and osmosis are passive processes (i.e., they do not require energy from body cells). The natural tendency of molecules or ions is to move from areas of high concentratrion to areas of lesser concentration. In diffusion the molecules move to areas of lesser solute concentration, and in osmosis the molecules move to areas with less solvent.[5] An active transport system moves molecules or ions "uphill" against concentration and osmotic pressure. The energy for active transport is supplied by metabolic process in the cells. Substances that are actively transported through the cell membrane include ions of sodium, potassium, calcium, iron, and hydrogen, some of the sugars, and the amino acids. An example of an active transport substance is insulin, which provides for transport of glucose from the extracellular compartment into the cell. We might liken the active transport system to a ski lift hauling skiers up a mountainside and then returning for more after dropping them at the top. Active transport systems exist for all the improtant electrolytes. Thus while solutes may move by diffusion and solvents by osmosis from areas of high concentration to areas of low concentration, substances may be moved in the opposite direction by the active transport system.

When an ion moves through a membrane from an area where it is less concentrated to an area where it is

active transport   more concentrated, a/an _____ system is required.

72 We have considered the movement of fluids and electrolytes in the body by diffusion, osmosis, and active transport. Another factor that influences the movement of fluids and electrolytes is *hydrostatic pressure.* Hydrostatic pressure is the force of fluid pressing outward against the vessel wall. When we relate hydrostatic pressure to the blood, we are referring not only to the pressure of the weight of the fluid against the wall of the capillary, but also to the force with which the blood is propelled by each heartbeat. Because of the force of the blood pressure, the hydrostatic pressure at the arterial end of the capillary is approximately twice as great as at the venous end.

arterial   Hydrostatic pressure is greater at the (arterial? venous?) end of the capillary.

73 When there is a difference in the hydrostatic pressure on two sides of a membrane, water and diffusible solutes move out of the solution that has the higher hydrostatic pressure. We call this process *filtration.*

The process by which water and solutes pass through a membrane when the hydrostatic pressure is greater on one side of the membrane than on the other is called

filtration   _____.

74 This tells us that hydrostatic pressures cause fluid and solutes, including nutrients, to be pushed out at the arterial end of the capillary.

Hydrostatic pressure in the arterial end of the capil-
leaving the capillary   lary results in fluid and solutes _____
(being pushed out)   _____.

75 Since there is fluid in the interstitial space, there is also hydrostatic pressure in the interstitial space from the weight of the fluid. However, the hydrostatic pressure is greater inside the arterial end of the capillary (because of the heartbeat) than is the interstitial hydrostatic pressure. Therefore fluid moves out of the capillary and into the interstitial space.

Fluid moves out of the capillary at the arterial end and into the interstitial tissue because of the difference in _____ pressure.

hydrostatic

76 We established earlier that this movement of fluid and diffusible solutes (those the capillary will allow through) is called *filtration*.

Filtration is the movement of fluid through a selectively permeable membrane from an area with higher hydrostatic pressure to an area with _____ hydrostatic pressure.

lower

77 If the hydrostatic pressure at the arterial end of a capillary is 37 mm Hg and the hydrostatic pressure of the interstitial fluid is 1 mm Hg, the resultant difference, or pressure gradient, will be 36 mm Hg and fluid will be pushed out of the capillary.

Therefore fluid will move (out of? into?) the arterial end of the capillary.

out of

78 However, we must remember that osmotic pressure also affects the movement of fluid between the intravascular and interstitial compartments. Remember: osmosis is the movement of solvent molecules across a selectively permeable membrane, and osmotic pressure (or pull) is determined by the number of particles of solute on the concentrated side. The osmotic pressure due to plasma colloids, or solutes, is called the *colloid osmotic* pressure or *oncotic* pressure.

Oncotic pressure is the osmotic pressure that is due to plasma _____.

solutes or colloids

79 Turn back to page 13 and look at the difference in the protein content between the intravascular and interstitial fluid.

intravascular The larger amount of protein is in the (intravascular? interstitial?) fluid.

80 This tells us that the oncotic pressure, or pull, will
into tend to move fluids (into? out of?) the capillary or intra-vascular compartment.

81 Let us look at the result of these two forces, hydro-static pressure and oncotic pressure, when we have both of them in the same place. At the arterial end of the capillary, the hydrostatic pressure is pushing water and solutes out, whereas the oncotic pressure is pulling water in. If the blood has an oncotic pressure of 26 mm Hg and the interstitial fluid an oncotic pressure of 1 mm Hg, the oncotic pressure gradient will be 25 mm Hg. The hydro-static pressure gradient will be 36 mm Hg, and the on-cotic pressure gradient will be 25 mm Hg, resulting in an 11 mm Hg pressure difference, which will cause fil-tration, or movement out of the arterial capillary.

Arterial end of capillary—hydrostatic pressure

Blood hydrostatic pressure	37 mm Hg
Interstitial fluid hydrostatic pressure	− 1 mm Hg
Hydrostatic pressure gradient	36 mm Hg

Arterial end of capillary—osmotic pressure

Blood osmotic (oncotic) pressure	26 mm Hg
Interstitial fluid osmotic pressure	− 1 mm Hg
Osmotic pressure gradient	25 mm Hg

Thus

Filtration force = Hydrostatic pres-sure gradient	36 mm Hg
Osmotic force = Osmotic pressure gradient	− 25 mm Hg
Net filtration force	11 mm Hg

greater **a** The blood hydrostatic pressure is (greater? less?) than the interstitial fluid hydrostatc pressure.
greater **b** The blood osmotic pressure is (greater? less?) than the interstitial fluid osmotic pressure.
greater **c** The filtration force is (greater? less?) than the osmotic force.
out of **d** The result is that water and solutes move (into? out of?) the capillary at the arterial end.

82 We shall now move over to the venous end of the capillary. In frame 72 we established that the hydrostatic pressure is about half as great at the venous end of the capillary as it is at the arterial end. We have the following situation at the venous end:

Venous end of capillary—hydrostatic pressure

Blood hydrostatic pressure	17 mm Hg
Interstitial fluid hydrostatic pressure	− 1 mm Hg
Hydrostatic pressure gradient	16 mm Hg

Venous end of capillary—osmotic pressure

Blood osmotic pressure	26 mm Hg
Interstitial fluid osmotic pressure	− 1 mm Hg
Osmotic pressure gradient	25 mm Hg

Thus

Osmotic force	25 mm Hg
Filtration force	− 16 mm Hg
Net osmotic pressure	9 mm Hg

a At the venous end the blood hydrostatic pressure is (greater? less?) than the osmotic force.

less

b The result is that at the venous end of the capillary, water and solutes move (into? out of?) the capillary.

into

Because of hydrostatic pressure and osmotic pressure, fluid and selected solutes move out of the capillary at the arterial end, whereas fluid and some solutes move into the capillary at the venous end.

Fluids and solutes enter the capillary at the venous end because of _____ pressure.

osmotic (oncotic)

83 About nine tenths of the fluid that filters out of the capillary at the arterial end is resorbed at the venous end. The other tenth of the fluid is returned to the vascular system by the lymph channels. The lymphatics can carry proteins and large particulate matter, which cannot be absorbed directly into the venous capillary, away from the tissue spaces. The permeability of the capillary wall varies in different parts of the body. For example, the capillaries in the liver allow protein through their membrane, whereas the capillaries in the renal glomeruli normally do not allow protein through their walls.

Capillary walls differ in permeability to (solutes? solvents?).

solutes

84 One example of a disturbance in the movement of fluids is in persons with pump failure (congestive heart failure) that goes on to pulmonary edema. In this situation the hydrostatic pressure in the lungs becomes severely increased. The hydrostatic pressure is increased so much that it overrides or exceeds the colloid osmotic pressure in the capillaries. The result is that large amounts of fluid from the capillaries move into the interstitial spaces in the lung.

a When the hydrostatic pressure in the capillaries exceeds the colloid osmotic pressure, fluid moves (into? out of?) the capillaries.

out of

b When the hydrostatic pressure exceeds the colloid osmotic pressure in the capillaries, fluid moves into the (capillaries? interstitial spaces?).

interstitial spaces

SUMMARY

Throughout the body the cell membranes and capillary walls are selectively permeable. Water and some solutes pass through the barrier freely, whereas other solutes require an active transport system.

Diffusion is the process by which a solute may spread throughout a solution. Molecules of a substance dissolved in a solvent spread by diffusion from an area of higher concentration to an area of lower concentration.

Osmosis is the movement of solvent molecules across a selectively permeable membrane to an area where there is a lesser concentration of solvent that can pass through the membrane. Since the solute cannot go through the membrane, the solvent moves to the area of lesser solvent concentration. The result of osmosis is two solutions, separated by a membrane, that are more nearly equal in concentration.

Osmotic pressure is the force that draws the solvent from a solution with more solvent activity through a selectively permeable membrane to a solution with less solvent activity. The amount of osmotic pressure is determined by the relative number of particles of solute on the side of greater concentration. When the solutions on each side of a selectively permeable membrane are equal in concentration, they are isotonic. A hypotonic solution has less solute than an isotonic solution, whereas a hypertonic solution contains more solute. If the selectively permeable membrane will allow the solvent to pass through but will not allow the solute through freely, the solvent will move to the side of greater solute concentration. If an ion is to move through a membrane from an area of low concentration to an area of high concentration, an active transport system is necessary.

Osmolality refers to the number of osmotically active particles per kilogram of water. In the body osmotic pressure is measured in milliosmoles. The normal osmolality of plasma is 280 to 294 mosm/kg.

Hydrostatic pressure is the force of the fluid pressing outward against some surface. When there is a difference in the hydrostatic pressure on two sides of a membrane, water and diffusible solutes move out of the solution that has the higher hydrostatic pressure. This process is called *filtration*. At the arterial end of the capillary, the hydrostatic pressure is greater than the osmotic pressure. Therefore fluid and diffusible solutes move out of the capillary. At the venous end the osmotic pressure, or pull, is greater than the hydrostatic pressure, and fluids and some solutes move into the capillary. The excess fluid and solutes remaining in the interstitial space are returned to the intravascular compartment by the lymph channels.

REVIEW

1 The process by which particles spread in all directions through a solution is called _____.

diffusion

2 The movement of fluid through a selectively permeable membrane is called _____.

osmosis

3 The force that draws solvent from a solution with more solvent through a selectively permeable membrane into a solution with less solvent is called _____

osmotic pressure

_____.

4 When the solutions on both sides of a selectively permeable membrane are alike in concentration, they are _____.

isotonic

5 If cells are placed in a hypotonic solution, they will

swell; burst _____ and may _____.

6 The process by which water and solutes pass through a membrane when the hydrostatic pressure is greater on one side of the membrane than on the other is called

filtration _____.

7 Water and some solutes move out of the capillary at the arterial end because the hydrostatic pressure gradient

osmotic is greater than the _____ pressure gradient.

8 At the venous end, water and some solutes move into the capillary because the filtration force is less than the

osmotic (oncotic) _____ force.

NORMAL MECHANISM BY WHICH WATER AND ELECTROLYTES ENTER AND LEAVE THE BODY

85 Normally water enters the body through three sources: oral liquids, water in foods, and water formed by oxidation of foods. Electrolytes are present in both foods and liquids. With a normal diet, an excess of essential electrolytes is taken in and the unused electrolytes are excreted.

Water is taken into the body through three sources. They are

oral liquids **a** _____

water in foods **b** _____

oxidation of foods **c** _____

86 The typical amount of intake for an adult is as follows:

Ingested liquids	1500 ml
Water in foods	700 ml
Water from oxidation	200 ml
TOTAL	2400 ml

The largest quantity of water is taken into the body

oral (ingested) liquids as _____.

87 Infants ingest and excrete a greater amount of fluid per kilogram of body weight than do older children or

28

Table 1. Calculation of maintenance fluids in children

Child's weight	Kilogram body weight formula
0-72 hr old	60-100 ml/kg
0-10 kg	100 ml/kg (may increase up to 150 ml if renal and cardiac function adequate)
11-20 kg	1000 ml for the first 10 kg + 50 ml for each kg over 10 kg
21-30 kg	1500 ml for the first 20 kg + 25 ml/kg for each kg over 20 kg

From Hazinski MF: Nursing care of the critically ill child, ed 2, St. Louis, 1991 Mosby–Year Book, Inc.

adults. An infant at age 3 months who weighs 5.4 kg requires 140 to 160 ml/kg, or 750 to 850 ml of fluid, over a 24-hour period. At age 6 months, an infant who weighs 7.3 kg requires 130 to 135 ml/kg, or 950 to 1100 ml of fluid, over a 24-hour period.[12]

more

a Infants need (more? less?) fluid per kilogram of body weight than do adults.

130

b At 6 months of age, an infant may require (100? 130? 170?) ml of fluid per kilogram of body weight over a 24-hour period.

88 While an infant requires 130 to 160 ml/kg of fluid over a 24-hour period, an adult requires approximately 30 ml of fluid per kilogram of body weight over a 24-hour period.

less than

The fluid needs of an adult are (more than? less than? the same as?) those of an infant.

89 Fluids leave the body by several routes. One way is through the skin. Water is lost through the skin of an adult by diffusion in the amount of 300 to 400 ml/day. The amount of water lost by diffusion through the skin is obligatory (i.e., it will be lost regardless of intake). We are not aware of losing water in this way through the skin; therefore it is called *insensible* perspiration.

300 to 400 (350)

The amount of water lost through the skin by diffusion is about _____ ml/day.

90 Water is also lost through the skin by perspiration—a process that we are aware of. The amount of water lost by perspiration will vary depending on the temperature of the environment and of the body. The average amount of water lost by perspiration in an adult is 100 ml/day. This amount may be increased to as much as 1.5 to 3.5 L/hr.

The usual amount of water lost by perspiration in an adult is _____ ml/day.

100

91 We are unaware of losing fluid through expired air, which is saturated with water vapor. The amount of water lost from the lungs will vary with the rate and depth of respirations. The average amount of water lost from the lungs in an adult is 300 to 400 ml/day. The water lost from the lungs and through the skin by diffusion is called insensible loss because we are unaware of losing that water.

In an adult the total average amount of water that we say is an insensible loss would be (100? 350? 700?) ml/day.

700

92 Large quantities of fluid are secreted into the gastrointestinal tract, but almost all of this fluid is resorbed. The average amount of water lost in the feces of an adult is 200 ml/day—equal to the amount of water gained through the oxidation of foods.

The normal amount of water lost through the feces of an adult is _____ ml/day.

200

93 A very large volume of electrolyte-containing liquid moves into the gastrointestinal tract and then returns again to the extracellular fluid. In an adult this amount is about 8000 ml/day. Since 8000 ml is such an enormous volume, we can understand the importance of any abnormal loss of gastrointestinal secretions. Severe diarrhea will result in the loss of large quantities of fluids and electrolytes.

An abnormal loss of secretions from the gastrointestinal tract is (serious? unimportant?).

serious

94 The organs that play a major role in regulating fluid and electrolyte balance are the kidneys. More than any other organ in the body, normal kidneys can adjust the amount of water and electrolytes leaving the body. The quantity of fluid excreted by the kidneys is determined by the amount of water ingested and the amount of waste or solutes excreted. The usual quantity of urine output for an adult is approximately 1400 ml/day. However, this will vary greatly, depending on fluid intake, amount of perspiration, and several other factors.

a The major organs that regulate fluid and electrolyte
kidneys   balance are the _____.
1400   **b** The usual quantity of urine for an adult is _____
ml/day.

95 An infant's kidneys are immature and are unable to concentrate or dilute urine. Therefore an infant requires more water and has difficulty conserving body water.

more   An infant requires (more? less? the same amount of?) water per kilogram of body weight than does an adult.

96 The amount of urine excreted in a 24-hour period depends on fluid intake, state of health, and age. The average amount of urine output for an infant at the age of 6 months is about 450 ml in 24 hours.

a At the age of 6 months, a healthy infant excretes ap-
450   proximately _____ ml of urine in 24 hours.
500;700   **b** Refer to "Urine Output" on p. 93 to see that a child excretes approximately _____ to _____ ml of urine in 24 hours.

97 The average total amount of water taken into the body by all three sources is 2400 ml/day in an adult. Average total amount of water leaving the body in an adult is:

Skin by diffusion	350 ml
Skin by perspiration	100 ml
Lungs	350 ml
Feces	200 ml
Kidneys	1400 ml
TOTAL	2400 ml

As long as all organs are functioning normally, the body is able to maintain balance in its fluid content.

2400

The average total output of water from all sources is _____ ml/day for an adult.

TYPES OF IMBALANCE

We shall now discuss three types of imbalance. There may be an imbalance in the volume, in the concentration, or in the composition of body fluids.

Fluid volume

98 In the diagram below, A, B, C, and D are electrolytes. Note the levels of volume.

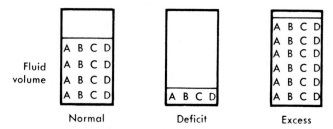

is no

volume

a There is a deficit in volume in the middle figure of this diagram. There (is? is no?) change in the concentration or composition of the electrolytes in the fluid in this figure.

b There is an excess of _____ in the third figure.

Fluid concentration

99 Besides an imbalance in the volume of fluid, another kind of imbalance is a change in the concentration of electrolytes in the fluid.

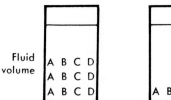

32

In the preceding diagram we have variations in the concentration of electrolytes in the three figures while the volume remains the same.

a The ratio of water to electrolytes in the middle figure is (increased? decreased?).

increased

b The volume has (increased? not changed? decreased?).

not changed

c The amount of electrolyte A in each figure is (more than? equal to? less than?) the amount of electrolyte B in the same figure.

equal to

d The volume is the same in each figure. The concentration is (the same? different?).

different

Fluid composition

100 We shall now look at variations in composition.

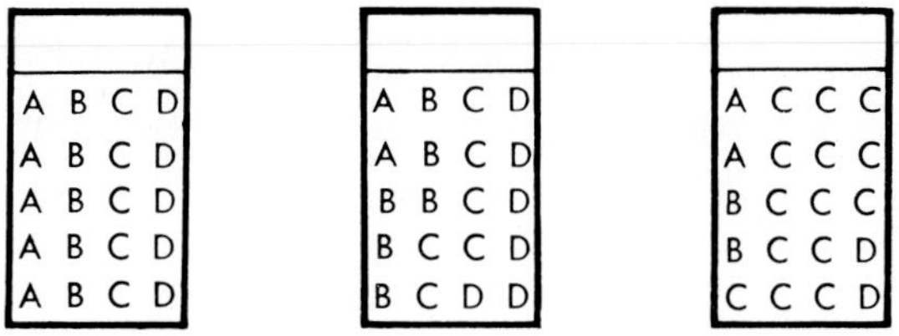

In each figure of the diagram the volume and the concentration of electrolytes are the same. The composition of electrolytes is different.

a In the left-hand figure the concentration of electrolytes A, B, C, and D is (equal? not equal?).

equal

b In the middle figure there is a deficit of electrolyte _____.

A

c In the right-hand figure there is an excess of electrolyte _____.

C

SUMMARY

The electrolyte composition of extracellular fluid is different from that of intracellular fluid. Sodium is the chief cation of extracellular fluid; potassium is the major

33

cation of intracellular fluid. At the arterial end of the capillary, hydrostatic pressure in the intravascular compartment is greater than osmotic pressure. Therefore some fluid moves out of the blood vessel. At the venous end of the capillary, fluid is drawn into the vessel because the osmotic pull is not counteracted by hydrostatic pressure. Hypertonic extracellular fluid causes the cells to shrink. Fluids cross the cell membrane by means of hydrostatic pressure and osmotic pressure. Electrolytes are transported across the cell membrane. An imbalance may occur in the volume, concentration, or composition of the fluid. If a person is to remain healthy, the fluids and electrolytes must be in balance.

REVIEW

1 The unit of measure that expresses the chemical combining power of an electrolyte is a _____.

milliequivalent

2 Fluids shift between the extracellular and the intracellular compartments by means of _____ _____ and _____.

hydrostatic pressure
osmosis

3 In the presence of a hypotonic solution, a cell will _____ and then may _____.

swell; burst

4 An imbalance in the composition of extracellular fluid means _____ _____.

an excess or a deficit
of an electrolyte

CONTROLS FOR MAINTAINING FLUID AND ELECTROLYTE BALANCE

101 If a person is to remain healthy, the volume, concentration, and composition of fluids and electrolytes must be maintained within narrow limits. This is an extremely complex task when we consider the billions of cells in the body constantly pouring the products of chemical reactions into the extracellular fluid and withdrawing from it substances needed for specific cellular activities. What we take into the body as food and fluid contains a wide variety of materials. Some food contains electrolytes at a concentration far in excess of levels permissible in body fluid. The volume of liquids we drink might drown us were there no mechanisms for maintaining constant volume of body fluid. These needs for maintaining balance, or homeostasis, are multiplied in disease.

The volume, concentration, and composition of body fluids must be _____.

kept within limits

102 We use the term *homeostasis* to indicate the relative stability of the internal environment. The composition of the internal environment may vary from tissue to tissue because of differences in cell activity and metabolism. Yet, because of the movement of substances between the compartments, a relative constancy is maintained. We recognize, then, that the internal environment is not static but is dynamic.

Homeostasis implies (stagnation? variation within limits?).

variation within limits

103 The maintenance of homeostasis depends on a variety of processes. Substances that the cells need must be available in adequate quantity. Some of the substances required by the cell are oxygen, water, a variety of nutrients including calories, tissue-building materials, and electrolytes. The intake, storage, and elimination of the substances must be maintained within safe limits. In health the body is able to respond to disturbances in fluids and electrolytes so as to prevent or repair damage. Thirst, the conscious desire for water, is one of the major factors that determine fluid intake. The osmoreceptors in the hypothalamus are cells that are stimulated by an increase in the osmotic pressure of body fluids to initiate thirst. After eating potato chips you become thirsty because the salt on the chips increased the osmotic pressure of body fluids.

a In a healthy person one of the factors that regulate fluid intake is _____.

thirst

b When the osmotic pressure of the body fluids increases, the _____ in the hypothalamus are stimulated to initiate thirst.

osmoreceptors

104 Thirst is also stimulated by a decrease in the extracellular fluid volume. This is another way in which the body attempts to regain balance—by increasing the intake of fluids.

A decrease in the volume of extracellular fluid will

thirst

stimulate _____.

105 Another factor that helps to regulate water intake is dryness of the mouth due to decreased salivary secretion. However, a person who has no deficit in fluid volume will become thirsty if given atropine, a drug that prevents salivation. A dry mouth does stimulate thirst but is not necessarily limited to decreased fluid intake. In a sick person the usual stimuli may be absent or inadequate. In a healthy person, thirst is stimulated by

increased

decreased

dry

a (increased? decreased?) osmotic pressure
b (increased? decreased?) extracellular fluid volume
c (dry? moist?) mucous membranes in the mouth

106 Homeostasis of the volume of water in the body is maintained or restored by adjusting the output to the intake. The kidneys carry the major responsibility to maintain balance of both fluids and electrolytes by controlling output. They are master chemists and remove waste materials or excessive substances from the extracellular fluid. The volume of urine is regulated primarily by hormones from the posterior lobe of the pituitary gland (antidiuretic hormone) and the adrenal cortex (aldosterone). These hormones will be discussed later. Influenced by these hormones, the kidneys help to regulate the total volume of extracellular fluids, the ratio of water to solutes (concentration), and the specific quantity of the different electrolytes (composition). When the extracellular fluid volume becomes too high, the blood volume, or intravascular volume, is increased. Therefore the venous return to the heart is increased, which then increases the cardiac output. This results in an increased arterial pressure. The increased arterial pressure resulting from the increased fluid volume causes the kidneys to excrete the excess fluid.

When the volume of extracellular fluid is too high, the

more

kidneys respond by excreting (more? less?) urine.

107 Normally the interstitial fluid volume is regulated so as to keep the interstitial fluid spaces filled. However, when this balance is not possible because of disease, the interstitial spaces can be expanded with excess fluid. Excess fluid in the interstitial spaces is called *edema*.

Edema is the result of increased fluid in the _____ _____ spaces.

interstitial

108 When the extracellular fluid volume is decreased because of increased loss or inadequate intake, the kidneys respond by retaining more fluid, so the extracellular fluid volume is returned to more nearly normal. However, if the extracellular fluid volume deficit is too great, the complex mechanisms affecting the kidney may not be enough to correct the imbalance, and treatment becomes necessary.

When the extracellular fluid volume is decreased, the kidneys respond by excreting (more? less?) urine.

less

109 Two hormonal systems play major roles in regulating fluid volume. One of these is the aldosterone system. Aldosterone is a hormone secreted by the adrenal cortex that regulates the extracellular volume by affecting the renal control of sodium and potassium.

The hormone from the adrenal cortex that affects extracellular fluid volume is _____.

aldosterone

110 When the adrenal glands are overactive or the production of aldosterone is increased, sodium, chloride, and water are retained in excessive amounts. However, large amounts of potassium are excreted. Thus aldosterone affects the renal excretion or retention not only of water, but also of some electrolytes.

a When there is an increased production of aldosterone, the kidneys retain (more? less?) sodium, chloride, and water.

more

b At the same time an increased production of aldosterone causes a (loss? gain?) of potassium.

loss

111 Aldosterone production is a complex and not completely understood mechanism. In a healthy person an increased production of aldosterone occurs when there is low fluid volume, low blood sodium, and high blood potassium.

Although the excretion or retention of sodium,

chloride, potassium, and water occurs through the kidneys, one of the hormones affecting this regulation is

aldosterone _____.

112 In a healthy person the production of aldosterone is controlled to maintain a balance of fluids and electrolytes in the body. If, because of disease, the adrenal glands become overactive and secrete more aldosterone than needed for homeostasis, a serious imbalance may occur. Various diseases of the adrenal glands result in overproduction of aldosterone. Cushing's syndrome is one disease in which the adrenal glands are overactive.

You would expect the symptoms to be the result of

potassium   **a** excretion of _____

sodium; chloride   **b** retention of _____, _____,

water   and _____.

113 If the adrenal glands become extremely underactive, the excretion of potassium will be decreased or more potassium will be retained in the body. Also, the level of sodium, chloride, and water will go down because these ions are lost from the body in the urine. There are various diseases in which the adrenal glands are hypoactive.

A person whose adrenal glands are very underactive

large   will excrete a (large? normal? small?) amount of urine.

114 We have looked briefly at some ways the kidneys are influenced by the hormone aldosterone to control the volume of extracellular fluid. Another hormone that affects extracellular fluid is the antidiuretic hormone (ADH). ADH is secreted by the posterior pituitary gland. Its name explains its action, *anti-* meaning against and *-diuretic* meaning increased secretion of urine. We could say that ADH is the water-conservation hormone. It regulates the osmotic pressure of extracellular fluid by regulating the amount of water resorbed from the blood by the renal tubules.

The hormone that is secreted by the posterior pituitary

ADH (antidiuretic hormone)   gland and that acts to conserve fluid is _____.

115 The ADH mechanism is complex, but the results of the action of ADH can be summarized. If there is an increased production of ADH, there will be increased amounts of water resorbed by the kidney through osmosis. The urine volume will be decreased, but the concentration will be increased.

The result of increased production of ADH is (increased? decreased?) volume of urine.

decreased

116 The usual stimulus to the production of ADH is an increase in the osmotic pressure of the extracellular fluids. ADH stimulates a retention of fluid to correct this increase in osmotic pressure. For example, if a large amount of hypertonic glucose solution is infused into the body, the osmotic pressure of the extracellular fluid will be increased. This will stimulate the production of more ADH, so more fluid will be retained and the osmotic pressure of the extracellular fluid will be returned to normal.

ADH production is regulated by changes in _____ pressure.

osmotic

117 For health to be maintained, the volume, concentration, and composition of body fluids and electrolytes must be kept within narrow limits. The regulation of these factors depends on intake and excretion.

Regulation of the loss of water and electrolytes depends primarily on the kidneys, which are affected by the hormones _____ and _____.

ADH; aldosterone

EXAMPLES OF FLUID AND ELECTROLYTE IMBALANCE

We have looked at three types of imbalance: volume, concentration, and composition. We can now talk about each separately, but we must remember that most patients will have a *combination* of imbalances.

Extracellular fluid volume imbalance

118 This type of imbalance may be a deficit in the volume of fluid without significant changes in electrolyte concentration. A deficit can be caused by an abrupt reduction in fluid intake, as when a patient is to take "nothing by mouth" (NPO). When a person is ill, there are times when neither food nor fluid is given by mouth. This may be in preparation for an anesthetic, or it may be to avoid stimulating the gastrointestinal tract. The signs and/or symptoms the nurse should look for in assessing fluid volume deficit include depression of the central nervous system (evidenced by reduced energy or stupor), depression of gastrointestinal activity with or without vomiting, reduced blood volume and flow of blood that leads to exhaustion, dry mucous membranes, and increased body temperature. In the treatment of extracellular fluid volume deficit without a significant change in the electrolyte concentration, fluids with electrolytes resembling the electrolytes in normal extracellular fluid are given. If the patient cannot be given fluids orally, the physician would order fluids to be given parenterally (e.g., by intravenous infusion).

A patient who is to take nothing by mouth will have

fluid volume

a deficit of _____.

fluids with electrolytes similar to those in normal extracellular fluid

119 In the treatment of a patient who has a deficit in fluid volume, the following are given: _____
_____
_____

Extracellular fluid concentration imbalance

120 A deficit in electrolyte concentration can occur in a patient who has a nasogastric tube in his stomach connected to suction. The patient will lose both fluids and electrolytes, especially sodium and potassium. In the treatment of this patient, fluids containing electrolytes would be ordered by the physician to restore the normal balance of both fluids and electrolytes. If the nasogastric tube is irrigated with water, even more electrolytes will be washed out. Therefore the tube must be irrigated only enough to keep it patent, or open. An isotonic solution such as normal saline (0.85% sodium chloride) should be used for irrigation.

A patient who has a nasogastric tube connected to suction will lose water and especially the electrolytes,

sodium; potassium

_____ and _____.

Imbalance in the composition of extracellular fluid

121 An example of an imbalance in the composition of electrolytes in body fluid is a deficit in potassium. A deficit in potassium can occur in infants who have diarrhea, in adults with ulcerative colitis, in burn patients who are healing, and in other conditions. Normally, when potassium (in very small quantities) moves out of the cell, sodium replaces it. This activity causes an electrochemical impulse to be transmitted along the nerve and muscle fibers. If potassium is not available in the cell, activating impulses are not transmitted to the muscles or nerves. The nurse should assess for neuromuscular depression that may progress to coma. There is depression of the gastrointestinal tract with paralytic ileus (absence of peristalsis). The muscles become soft, and the electrocardiogram will show changes when the potassium deficit becomes severe and the heart cannot continue to beat.

potassium

a Activating impulses are not transmitted to the muscles or nerves when _____ is not available in the cell.

potassium

b The major cation in the intracellular fluid is _____ .

122 When potassium has been lost from the cell because of the depletion of potassium in the extracellular fluid, several days of therapy may be needed to restore the depleted intracellular stores. Potassium may be given orally or parenterally. Remember: the exchange of fluids between the intravascular and interstitial spaces occurs rapidly through the capillary. By comparison, the rate of exchange of electrolytes across the cell membrane is slow.

days

If potassium is depleted in the extracellular fluid to the extent that the intracellular potassium becomes low, (minutes? hours? days?) of therapy may be required to restore the intracellular potassium level.

123 Since potassium is one of the ions necessary for the transmission of impulses to muscles and nerves, a severe deficit in potassium that is not corrected can be serious.

Death may result from weakness of the respiratory muscles and myocardial failure.

a deficit

Death may result from weakness of the respiratory muscles and myocardial failure when there is (a deficit? an excess?) of potassium.

a deficit

SUMMARY

The volume, concentration, and composition of body fluids must remain nearly constant. The kidneys play a major role in controlling all types of balance in fluids and electrolytes. The adrenal glands, through secretion of aldosterone, also aid in controlling extracellular fluid volume by regulating the amount of sodium resorbed by the kidneys. ADH, from the pituitary gland, regulates the osmotic pressure of extracellular fluid by regulating the amount of water resorbed by the kidneys. Remember: almost any patient who has an imbalance of fluids or electrolytes will have a combination of imbalances. When one of the substances (fluids or electrolytes) is deficient, it must be replaced either normally by intake of food and water or by medical therapy—such as intravenous infusions and/or medication. When there is an excess of fluids or electrolytes, therapy is directed toward helping the body to eliminate the excess.

REVIEW

excess fluid in interstitial spaces

1 Edema is the result of _____.

kidneys

2 The organs primarily responsible for the regulation of volume, concentration, and composition of body fluids are the _____.

sodium
potassium

3 A person who has gastric suction or has had prolonged vomiting will have a deficit of water, _____, and _____.

a combination

4 The type of imbalance most likely to occur in a patient is _____.

PART 2 Acid-base balance/imbalance

HYDROGEN ION CONCENTRATION

124 *Acid-base balance* means homeostasis of the hydrogen ion concentration in body fluids. Even a slight deviation in the hydrogen ion concentration causes pronounced changes in the rate of chemical reactions. Therefore survival is threatened when the hydrogen ion concentration deviates from normal. An increase in concentration of hydrogen ions (H^+) makes a solution more acidic; a decrease makes it more alkaline. The amount of ionized hydrogen in the extracellular fluid is extremely small, approximately 0.0000001 gram per liter (g/L). The number 0.0000001 may be expressed mathematically as 10^{-7}. For convenience, the minus sign is dropped and this concentration (10^{-7}) of hydrogen ions is indicated as pH 7. The symbol pH may be translated as the *power of hydrogen*; therefore the p is lowercased and the H (the symbol for hydrogen) is capitalized. Since this is a negative logarithm (exponent) of the hydrogen ion concentration, a pH of 8 would be 0.00000001 (10^{-8}), or one-tenth pH 7. Therefore the pH value falls as the hydrogen ion concentration rises; and as the concentration falls, the pH rises. (Acidity increases with a decreasing pH and decreases with an increasing pH.) The hydrogen ion concentration in body fluids determines the degree of acidity or alkalinity.

a Acid-base balance of body fluids is determined by the

hydrogen ions

concentration of _____.

43

pH

b The symbol used to indicate the concentration of hydrogen ions is _____.

125 A solution is acidic, neutral, or alkaline, depending on the number of hydrogen ions present. When the number of hydrogen ions increases to a certain point, the fluid becomes acidic. We report the hydrogen ion concentration in terms of pH. *Acidity* increases as the *pH* value *decreases*.

acidic

A pH of 7.1 is more (acidic? alkaline?) than a pH of 7.6.

126 *Alkalinity* increases as the *pH* value *increases*. When hydrogen ion concentration rises, the pH value falls. Conversely, when the hydrogen ion concentration falls, the pH value increases.

alkaline

A pH of 7.5 is more (acidic? alkaline?) than a pH of 7.1.

127 An acid is a substance that can give hydrogen ions, or is a hydrogen ion donor. Hydrogen ions carry a positive electrical charge and are therefore protons. Hydrogen ions are indicated by the symbol H^+.

A substance that can give up, or donate, hydrogen ions is a/an _____.

acid

128 A substance that accepts hydrogen ions can be called a proton acceptor, or a base.

accepts

A base is a substance that (accepts? donates?) hydrogen ions.

129 Acids such as sulfuric and hydrochloric form solutions containing a high concentration of hydrogen ions when placed in water. Therefore they are regarded as strong acids. Carbonic and acetic acids are considered weak acids because in solution they provide a low concentration of hydrogen ions.

high

In solution a strong acid will release a (high? low?) concentration of hydrogen ions.

130 A base is a hydrogen ion (proton) acceptor. In solution a base or alkaline compound will form hydroxyl ions (OH^-).

accept

A base will (accept? give?) protons.

131 An acid will donate protons, whereas a base will accept protons. In solution a base will form hydroxyl ions (OH^-), and an acid will form hydrogen ions (H^+). One exception is ammonia (NH_3), which will accept protons to form NH_4 but will not form hydroxyl ions in solution.
a An acid will donate protons and in solution will yield

H^+ (hydrogen ions)

_____.

b A base will accept protons and therefore will carry a

negative

(negative? positive?) electrical charge.

132 A solution at pH 7 is neutral because at that concentration there are equal numbers of both hydrogen ions (H^+) and hydroxyl ions (OH^-), which combine to form water (H_2O). The H^+ and OH^- are completely balanced. An acidic solution has a pH value below 7; an alkaline solution has a pH value above 7. The extracellular fluid of the body is normally maintained within the range of pH 7.35 to 7.45.

alkaline
equal (balanced)

a The extracellular fluid is slightly (acidic? alkaline?).
b At pH 7 the H^+ and the OH^- are _____.

133 The extreme limits that are compatible with life are an arterial pH of about 6.8 to 7.9. In either extreme the imbalance may result in death if not corrected.

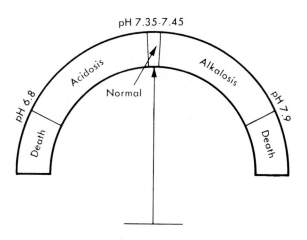

pH 7.35-7.45

alkalosis

At a pH of 7.5 the body is in a state of _____.

45

134 Refer to the diagram on page 45.

a If the body fluids have a pH of 7.2, the body is in a

acidosis   state of _____.

death   **b** If the pH goes below 6.8, _____ will occur.

135 When the pH goes below 7.35, some degree of acidosis exists because there is an increase in the concentration of hydrogen ions. As the pH becomes more acidic, the central nervous system is depressed and symptoms varying from disorientation to coma result.

depress   Acidosis, an increase in hydrogen ion concentration, will (depress? stimulate?) the central nervous system.

136 When the pH goes above 7.45, some degree of alkalosis is present because there is a decrease in the concentration of hydrogen ions. Alkalosis causes an overstimulation of the central nervous system. In alkalosis the nerve cells may generate impulses even without the normal stimuli; the symptoms may range from tingling sensations in the fingers and toes to convulsions.

stimulate   Alkalosis will (depress? stimulate?) the central nervous system.

137 Slight changes in hydrogen ion concentration from the narrow range of normal pH (7.35 to 7.45) cause marked changes in the rates of chemical reactions in the cells. Some chemical reactions are depressed, and others accelerated. This is the reason why regulation of the hydrogen ion concentration is one of the most important functions of the body. The more specific effects of changes in hydrogen ion concentration will be discussed throughout the remainder of Part 2. In general, when the body is in acidosis, the patient is likely to die in coma; when the body becomes alkalotic, he may die of tetany or convulsions.

a The normal range of pH in the extracellular fluids is

7.35 and 7.45   between _____.

b If the pH does not remain within these limits, the

increased   effect on cells will be one of _____ or

decreased   _____ chemical reactions.

46

c Severe acidosis as well as severe alkalosis will result

death

in _____ if the imbalance is not corrected.

138 We have been considering the pH or hydrogen ion concentration of extracellular fluid. Attempts have been made to measure intracellular pH. However, it is impossible to directly measure intracellular pH clinically for the purpose of treating an imbalance. The intracellular pH is generally lower than the extracellular pH, although it varies in different organs. Intracellular pH varies in a parallel direction with changes in the extracellular pH. Studies indicate that the intracellular pH value of cells may vary but is approximately 7 under normal conditions. When the pH is measured clinically, this represents hydrogen ion concentration in the extracellular fluid.

extracellular

Clinically the (extracellular? intracellular?) fluid is used in measuring pH.

SUMMARY

The concentration of hydrogen ions determines the acidity or alkalinity of body fluids. The hydrogen ion concentration is indicated by pH. At pH 7 the hydrogen ions and hydroxyl ions are balanced and the solution is neutral. The pH rises above 7 in an alkaline solution. An acidic solution has a pH below 7. The normal pH of body fluids is between pH 7.35 and 7.45. If the pH of body fluids goes beyond these limits, some chemical reactions in the body will be accelerated and others will be depressed. Either severe acidosis or alkalosis will result in death if not corrected.

REVIEW

1 The term used to indicate a measure of hydrogen ion

pH

concentration is _____.

neutral

2 A pH of 7 is _____.

acidic

3 A pH of 7.2 is more _____ than a pH of 7.5.

4 A pH of 7 represents ten times the concentration of hydrogen ions as does a pH of _____.

5 Slight changes in the hydrogen ion concentration outside the range of normal will cause a/an _____ or _____ rate of chemical reactions in some cells.

DEFENSE MECHANISMS

139 What determines the pH of extracellular fluid, and how is extracellular pH maintained? We shall discuss the pH of extracellular fluid because the pH of intracellular fluid is not measurable clinically (although intracellular pH does vary with extracellular pH). We know that the normal pH range in the body is 7.35 to 7.45. When the pH goes down, acidosis exists because there are more hydrogen ions available. In alkalosis the concentration of hydrogen ions is decreased. Normally the body maintains the pH between the narrow range of 7.35 and 7.45, even though it is constantly adding acids and bases from metabolism and from ingested food and fluids. To maintain acid-base balance, the body has three lines of defense: the buffer system, the respiratory system, and the renal system. The buffer system can act within a fraction of a second to prevent excessive changes in the hydrogen ion concentration. In 1 to 3 minutes the respiratory system working alone can readjust the concentration after a sudden change has occurred. Although the kidneys are the most powerful of the control mechanisms, if they are working alone, they will require from several hours to a day or more to readjust the hydrogen ion concentration after a sudden change. Each of the mechanisms shares the responsibility of maintaining normal hydrogen ion concentration.

The three mechanisms maintaining normal hydrogen ion concentration are

a _____

b _____

c _____

The buffer system

140 A buffer may be regarded as a chemical sponge. Depending on the circumstances, the sponge can soak up surplus hydrogen ions or release them. An acid-base buffer is a solution of two or more chemical compounds that prevents excessive changes in the hydrogen ion concentration when either an acid or a base is added to the solution. For example, if only a few drops of concentrated hydrochloric acid are added to a beaker of pure water (pH 7), the pH of the water may immediately fall as low as 1. However, if a satisfactory buffer is present, the hydrochloric acid will combine with the buffer and the pH will fall only slightly.

a The pH falls when the hydrogen ion concentration (increases? decreases?).

increases

b An acid-base buffer should prevent excessive changes in _____.

pH (hydrogen ion concentration)

141 There are a number of buffer systems in the body. However, the primary buffer system is the bicarbonate–carbonic acid system, also called the carbonate system, which consists of a mixture of carbonic acid (H_2CO_3) and sodium bicarbonate ($NaHCO_3$) in the same solution. Carbonic acid is a very weak acid; its degree of dissociation (into hydrogen ions and bicarbonate ions) is less than that of other acids. Most of the carbonic acid in solution dissociates into carbon dioxide and water, the net result being a high concentration of dissolved carbon dioxide but only a weak concentration of acid. Hydrolysis of bicarbonate in solution yields the hydroxyl ion and thus increases the alkalinity in the solution. Normally, to maintain acid-base balance (pH 7.35 to 7.45), the ratio of carbonic acid to base bicarbonate is 1:20.

$$\frac{H_2CO_3}{BHCO_3} = \frac{1}{20} = pH\ 7.4$$

There are also small amounts of potassium bicarbonate, calcium bicarbonate, and magnesium bicarbonate in the body. The symbol $BHCO_3$ is used to indicate any of these base bicarbonates.

a To maintain acid-base balance of body fluids, there

20

must be 1 part acid to _____ parts base in the carbonate buffer system.

b The primary buffer system in the body is the

carbonate

_____ system.

c Carbonic acid is a weak acid because most of it dis-

carbon dioxide

sociates into _____

water

and _____.

d An increased amount of available hydroxyl ions will

alkalinity

increase the (acidity? alkalinity?) of a solution.

142 When hydrochloric acid (HCl), a strong acid, is added to a solution containing sodium bicarbonate, the following reaction takes place:

$$HCl + NaHCO_3 \rightarrow H_2CO_3 + NaCl$$

weak

Instead of the strong hydrochloric acid, we have the (strong? weak?) carbonic acid (H_2CO_3).

143 Since the strong acid combines with the sodium bicarbonate to form a weak acid and sodium chloride, the hydrochloric acid that was added to the buffer solution

slightly

changes the pH (slightly? excessively?).

144 When a strong acid is added in the presence of a

slightly

buffer system, the pH decreases (slightly? greatly?).

145 If sodium hydroxide (NaOH), which is a strong base, is added to a buffer solution, the following reaction will occur:

$$NaOH + H_2CO_3 \rightarrow NaHCO_3 + H_2O$$

This shows that the hydroxyl ion of the sodium hydroxide combines with the hydrogen ion from the carbonic acid to form water and sodium bicarbonate.

weak

Sodium bicarbonate is a (strong? weak?) base.

146 If a strong base is added to a buffer solution, the pH

increase

will _____ only slightly.

147 There are four main buffer systems in the body that help to maintain the constancy of the pH. These major buffer systems are the bicarbonate–carbonic acid system, the phosphate system, the protein system, and the hemoglobin system. Although the carbonate buffer system is not especially powerful, it is as important as the combination of all the other buffer systems in the body because *each* of the two elements of the carbonate system can be regulated through carbon dioxide content by the respiratory system and through bicarbonate ion by the kidneys. The buffer system is one of the mechanisms the body has for regulating pH.

The most important buffer in the body is the

carbonate _____ system.

The respiratory system

148 Carbon dioxide is being formed continuously in the body by the different intracellular metabolic processes. For example, the carbon in foods is oxidized to form carbon dioxide. The carbon dioxide diffuses out of the cells and into the interstitial fluids and then into the intravascular fluids. Carbon dioxide is transported to the lungs, where it diffuses into the alveoli and is exhaled. If its rate of metabolic formation is increased, its concentration in the extracellular fluids will also be increased. If the rate of pulmonary ventilation (respirations) is increased, the rate of expiration of carbon dioxide will also be increased—which will lower the amount of accumulated carbon dioxide in the extracellular fluids.

a If metabolism decreases, the carbon dioxide concentration in body fluids will (increase? decrease?).

decrease

b If the respiratory rate is decreased, the amount of carbon dioxide in the extracellular fluids will (increase? decrease?).

increase

149 Because of the ability of the respiratory center to respond to the hydrogen ion concentration, which is the result of direct action by hydrogen ions on the respiratory center in the medulla, and because changes in respiratory ventilation in turn alter the hydrogen ion concentration in body fluids, the respiratory system acts as a feedback system for controlling hydrogen ion concentration. When the hydrogen ion concentration increases

51

(acidosis) in the extracellular fluids, the respiratory system becomes more active (increased rate and depth of respirations) and more carbon dioxide is exhaled. Therefore the carbon dioxide concentration in the extracellular fluids decreases. Since more carbon dioxide is removed, there is less available to combine with water to form carbonic acid.

$$H_2O + CO_2 \rightleftharpoons H_2CO_3 \rightleftharpoons H^+ + HCO_3^-$$

carbon dioxide

Less carbonic acid is formed when less _____ _____ is available. Therefore the pH does not fall as it would if more carbonic acid were present in the extracellular fluid.

less

150 When the hydrogen ion concentration decreases, the respiratory system becomes (more? less?) active and the carbon dioxide concentration increases.

carbonic acid

151 If more carbon dioxide is available, more _____ _____ will be formed.

152 The respiratory mechanism for regulation of hydrogen ion concentration has an efficiency of 50% to 75%. For example, if the pH suddenly drops from 7.4 to 7, the respiratory system will return the pH to about 7.2 to 7.3 within a minute. The reason for this level of efficiency is that as the hydrogen ion concentration approaches normal, the stimulus to the respiratory center is lost. Then the chemical buffering systems, which were discussed earlier, aid in achieving balance.

partially

The respiratory system is capable of returning the pH (partially? completely?) to normal.

The renal system

153 Since the kidneys can excrete varying amounts of acid or base, they play a vital role in the control of pH. The renal regulation of body pH is a complex device for excreting varying amounts of hydrogen ions from the body, depending on the number of hydrogen ions entering the blood. This involves a series of reactions that occur in the renal tubules, including reactions for hydrogen ion secretion, sodium ion resorption, bicarbonate ion excretion into the urine, and ammonia secretion into the tubules. The bicarbonate ion entering the renal tubules changes in proportion to the extracellular bicarbonate ion concentration. When the bicarbonate ion concentration in the extracellular fluid remains normal (see the diagram on page 57), the hydrogen ion secretion and bicarbonate ion filtration normally balance and neutralize each other.

The concentration of bicarbonate ions that enter the kidneys (varies? does not vary?).

varies

154 In normal metabolism the body produces an excess of acids. To maintain balance, the kidneys excrete more hydrogen ions, and therefore the urine is usually acidic.

When more hydrogen ions are excreted in the urine, the pH of urine becomes more (acidic? alkaline?).

acidic

155 Excess hydrogen ions are excreted in the urine.

When the bicarbonate ion concentration in the extracellular fluid is greater than normal, (more? less?) bicarbonate ions than are needed to combine with hydrogen ions enter the renal tubules.

more

156 When this happens, the excess _____ _____ are excreted by the kidneys in the urine.

bicarbonate ions

157 Though the kidneys are able to excrete either an alkaline or an acidic urine, the urine is usually acidic.

When more bicarbonate ions are excreted, the urine becomes more (acidic? alkaline?).

alkaline

158 Although the renal system acts slowly, it differs from the respiratory mechanism in that it continues to act until the extracellular pH reaches exactly normal. The elderly person has a decrease in nephrons in the kidney, which may then require more time for the renal system to achieve balance. A younger adult may need 6 to 10 hours to achieve acid-base balance, whereas in the elderly person it may take 18 to 48 hours.

a The respiratory mechanism for maintaining acid-base balance has an efficiency of 50% to 75%, but the renal

completely

more

system has the advantage of being able to neutralize (partially? completely?) the excess acid or alkali that enters body fluids.

b The renal system in an elderly person may require (more? same? less?) time to achieve acid-base balance than (as) that of a younger adult.

Summary of mechanisms for maintaining normal hydrogen ion concentration

The buffer system

Bicarbonate-carbonic acid (primary buffer system)	Carbonic acid (weak acid) $H_2CO_3 \rightleftharpoons H_2O + CO_2$
	Sodium bicarbonate (weak base) $NaHCO_3$
In the presence of a buffer system the pH shifts only slightly	$NaHCO_3 + HCl \rightarrow H_2CO_3 + NaCl$ (strong (weak acid) acid)
	$H_2CO_3 + NaOH \rightarrow NaHCO_3 + H_2O$ (strong (weak base) base)

The respiratory system

The respiratory system acts as a feedback system for controlling hydrogen ion concentration	H^+ concentration increases pH 7.4 → 7 Respirations →rapid and deep More CO_2 exhaled Less CO_2 to combine Therefore, less H_2CO_3
50% to 75% efficient	pH from 7 to 7.2 or 7.3 within minutes
	OR
	H^+ concentration decreases pH 7.4 → 7.8 Respirations → slow and shallow Less CO_2 exhaled More CO_2 to combine Therefore, more H_2CO_3
	pH from 7.8 to 7.6 or 7.7 within minutes

The renal system

This complex mechanism continues to act until the pH reaches normal; requires more time	Can excrete more or less H^+ to achieve balance Can excrete more or less bicarbonate to achieve balance

159 By returning some substances to body fluids and excreting others, the kidneys can compensate in several hours for even large deviations from the normal concentration of acid or base.

a If the pH of extracellular fluid goes down, the kidneys will eliminate more (hydrogen ions? bicarbonate ions?) to achieve balance.

hydrogen ions

b If the extracellular fluid pH goes up, the kidneys will eliminate more (hydrogen? bicarbonate?) ions to attain balance.

bicarbonate

SUMMARY

The homeostatic mechanisms we have considered are those that function to maintain electrolyte balance when a person is healthy. In illness the function of one of the regulating mechanisms may be affected, or the imbalance of either acid or base in the body may become too great for the body to correct without treatment.

The body has three mechanisms for the regulation of acid-base balance: the buffer system, the respiratory system, and the renal system.

The buffer system involves two or more compounds that prevent excessive changes in the pH of body fluids. The most important buffer is the bicarbonate–carbonic acid system. Carbonic acid is weak and ionizes to a limited extent.

$$H_2CO_3 \rightleftharpoons H^+ + HCO_3^-$$

Bicarbonate is a weak base and yields the hydroxyl ion.

$$HCO_3^- + H_2O \rightleftharpoons H_2CO_3 + OH^-$$

The pH of the extracellular fluid can be brought back to normal by this system.

The respiratory system helps to maintain acid-base balance through the control of carbon dioxide content. When the amount of carbon dioxide in the extracellular fluids increases, the respirations are increased in rate and depth to exhale more carbon dioxide. If the level of carbon dioxide is low, respirations are depressed. When more carbon dioxide is removed, there is less to combine with water to form carbonic acid.

The kidneys can eliminate either hydrogen ions or bicarbonate ions from body fluids and in this way can increase or decrease the pH. The renal mechanism requires more time than the other systems, but it is more powerful.

REVIEW

1 The defenses that the body has to maintain acid-base balance are

buffer system **a** _____

respiratory system **b** _____

renal system **c** _____

2 The most important chemical buffer system in the

carbonate system body is the _____.

3 When a strong acid is added in the presence of a buffer

decreased slightly system, the pH is _____.

4 When the hydrogen ion concentration in the extracellular fluid increases, the respiratory system becomes

more active _____.

5 When the bicarbonate concentration in the extracel-

excrete more lular fluids is greater than normal, the kidneys _____

bicarbonate ions _____.

CLINICAL CONDITIONS OF IMBALANCE

160 Any factor that decreases the rate of pulmonary ventilation will increase the concentration of dissolved carbon dioxide, carbonic acid, and hydrogen ions.

acidosis   The result of this process is (acidosis? alkalosis?).

Respiratory acidosis

161 Respiratory acidosis is caused by any clinical situation that interferes with pulmonary gas exchange and causes retention of carbon dioxide, resulting in an increase in the blood carbonic acid.

a For example, in emphysema (chronic obstructive pulmonary disease) there is obstruction to the exchange of oxygen and carbon dioxide that causes a retention of carbon dioxide, resulting in an increase of

carbonic acid

_____ in the extracellular fluid.

more

b The pH of the extracellular fluid becomes (more? less?) acid than normal.

162

a Normal balance

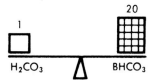

b Imbalance due to disease involving the lungs

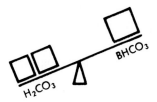

carbonic acid

Because of disease, carbon dioxide is retained in the body; thus there is more _____ in the extracellular fluids.

c To bring about balance, the kidneys conserve base

hydrogen ions

bicarbonate and excrete _____. The

acidic

urine then becomes _____.

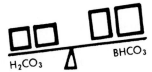

d If the body's regulating mechanisms succeed in maintaining balance, the acidosis will be compensated or corrected. If the imbalance cannot be corrected by the regulating mechanisms of the body, then medical therapy will be necessary. Treatment will be directed first at the cause (e. g., emphysema); then medication containing bicarbonate may be necessary. This usually involves solutions of sodium bicarbonate or lactate-containing solutions given intravenously. If sodium lactate is used, the lactate will be oxidized to carbonic acid, allowing the sodium to react with carbonic acid to form sodium bicarbonate. A mechanical respirator may be used to improve ventilation.

base

If the respiratory acidosis must be treated, the patient will need more (acid? base?).

163 In respiratory acidosis the problem or disease affects the respirations. Therefore the respiratory system is not available as a compensating or correcting factor.

more

The kidneys compensate by excreting (more? less?) hydrogen ions to return the pH to a normal level.

164 In respiratory acidosis the problem is excess carbonic acid that cannot be reduced by exhaling more carbon dioxide, since the respiratory system is affected by a pathological condition.

carbonic acid

Respiratory acidosis results from an excess of _____.

Respiratory alkalosis

165 In respiratory alkalosis the problem is the result of a lack of carbonic acid. Respiratory alkalosis does not occur as frequently as does respiratory acidosis.

carbon dioxide

Whenever there is excessive pulmonary ventilation of relatively normal lungs, there will be an increased loss of _____.

decrease

166 When excessive amounts of carbon dioxide are exhaled, there is a resultant (increase? decrease?) of carbonic acid in the extracellular fluid.

167 Respiratory alkalosis occurs when pulmonary ventilation is excessive and there is a decrease on the carbonic acid side of the carbonic acid-base bicarbonate ratio. Respiratory alkalosis occurs in hypoxia due to high altitude, encephalitis, or fever, because of the stimulation to the respiratory center. Salicylate poisoning, such as from an overdose of aspirin, also causes direct stimulation of the respiratory center.

The body attempts to return the pH to normal levels through the kidneys by excreting bicarbonate ions and

retaining

_____ hydrogen ions.

168

a Normal balance

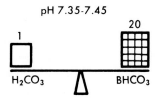

pH 7.35-7.45

H_2CO_3 $BHCO_3$

b Imbalance due to disease

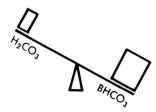

Respirations have increased, thus there is a loss of

carbon dioxide

_____.

c To bring about balance, the kidneys excrete bicarbonate ions and retain _____.

hydrogen ions

The urine is _____.

alkaline

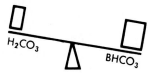

H_2CO_3 $BHCO_3$

d If the regulatory mechanism of the body cannot correct the imbalance, therapy will be directed at the cause. Included will be treatment to correct the original condition, such as the cause of a high fever. Next, carbon dioxide may be given by mask inhalation for brief intervals. Medications to increase the acid concentration will be ordered by the physician.

In compensating for the respiratory alkalosis, both the carbonic acid and the base bicarbonate levels are decreased. Treatment is aimed at increasing the (acid? base?) side.

acid

169 In respiratory alkalosis some factor has affected the respiratory system so that increased amounts of carbon dioxide are _____.

exhaled

a To compensate, the kidneys excrete _____ _____.

bicarbonate ions

carbon dioxide

b In the treatment _____ may be given by mask inhalation for short intervals.

Metabolic acidosis

170 Some clinical conditions that may lead to metabolic acidosis are severe diarrhea, vomiting, uremic acidosis, and diabetes mellitus. For example, in diabetes the lack of insulin prevents the use of glucose for metabolism. The stored fats are oxidized into acids. Acetoacetic acid is one of those acids and is metabolized for energy. The acetoacetic acid concentration in the extracellular fluids often rises to a very high level, and large quantities are excreted in the urine. Metabolic acidosis occurs because of the high acid content in extracellular fluid and also because the acetoacetic acid carries large quantities of sodium as sodium bicarbonate with it into the urine.

Metabolic acidosis results because of the high acid content of the blood, which also causes a loss of _____ _____, the alkaline half of the carbonate buffer system.

sodium bicarbonate

171
a Normal balance

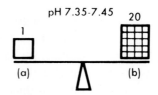

pH 7.35-7.45

(a)   (b)

H_2CO_3, $BHCO_3$

In the diagram on page 60, the labels should read (a) ____________ (b) ____________

b Diabetic acidosis (acetoacetic acid combines with bicarbonate)

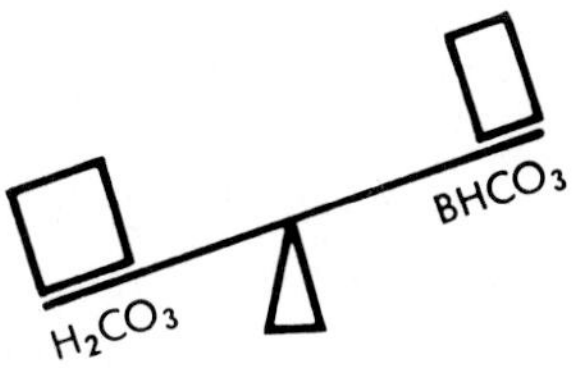

c Regulatory mechanisms

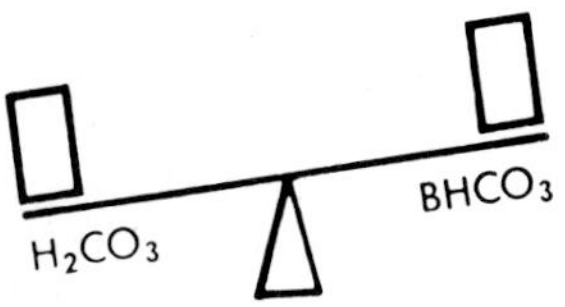

hyperactive (deep and rapid)

(1) Breathing becomes ____________ (Kussmaul breathing).

carbon dioxide

(2) The lungs exhale more ____________.

acidic

(3) The kidneys excrete hydrogen ions, and the urine becomes ____________.

d In metabolic acidosis there is usually an extracellular fluid volume deficit that must be corrected by parenteral fluids. To treat diabetic acidosis, carbohydrates and insulin must be supplied. Intravenous solutions of sodium bicarbonate or lactate (such as sodium lactate) may also be needed to support the base bicarbonate.

base bicarbonate

Treatment is aimed at correcting the cause of the metabolic acidosis and replacing the ____________ ____________ deficit.

base (alkali)

172 In metabolic acidosis there is a deficit in available ____________.

respiratory, renal, and buffer systems

a The homeostatic mechanisms that function to return the pH to a normal level include ____________ ____________.

hydrogen ions

b The kidneys excrete ____________.

7.35 to 7.45

173 The normal pH of the extracellular fluids is ____________ ____________.

174 In diabetic acidosis the respirations are called *Kussmaul breathing*. Since the respiratory system functions to return the pH to a more nearly normal level, the respirations become _____.

hyperactive
(deep and rapid)

Metabolic alkalosis

175 Metabolic alkalosis may be caused by ingestion of large amounts of sodium bicarbonate or by the loss of chloride through vomiting or gastric suction. When chloride is lost, the sodium that is left forms excessive sodium bicarbonate.

a Normal balance

7.35 to 7.45

   (1) Normal pH is _____.

Ratio of acid?	Ratio of base?

1:20

   (2) In the carbonate buffer system the ratio of acid to base is _____.

H_2CO_3

BHCO$_3$

   (3) The symbol for carbonic acid is _____ ; the symbol for base bicarbonate is _____.

increased

b Base bicarbonate is (increased? decreased?).

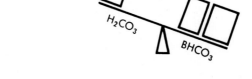

c Regulatory mechanisms

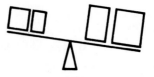

slow; shallow
retain
hydrogen ions
alkaline

(1) Breathing becomes _____ and _____, the lungs _____ carbon dioxide.

(2) The kidneys retain _____, causing the urine to become more _____.

d If the body's regulatory mechanisms cannot bring about balance, a chloride-containing solution will be given. The chloride ions of the solution promote excretion of the bicarbonate ions and help to relieve the base bicarbonate excess.

base bicarbonate

The major factor causing an imbalance in metabolic alkalosis is _____ excess.

conserving
carbon dioxide

176 The lungs help to return the pH to normal by _____.

Table 2. Summary of acid-base imbalance

Type	Etiology	Compensation
Respiratory acidosis (carbonic acid excess)	Chronic lung disease Surgery	Buffer system Renal system: excrete more H^+
Respiratory alkalosis (carbonic acid deficit)	Increased pulmonary ventilation Encephalitis Hypoxia Fever Salicylate poisoning	Buffer system Renal system: excrete more HCO_3^-
Metabolic acidosis (base deficit)	Diabetic ketoacidosis Uremic acidosis Diarrhea	Buffer system Respiratory system: rapid and deep Renal system: excrete more H^+, retain more HCO_3^-
Metabolic alkalosis (base excess)	Excessive ingestion of base (antacids) Vomiting Gastric suction	Buffer system Respiratory system: slow and shallow Renal system: retain more H^+, excrete more HCO_3^-

Combination of types of imbalance

177 We have considered respiratory acidosis and alkalosis and metabolic acidosis and alkalosis as separate entities. It is possible to have a combination of types of imbalance. For example, salicylates can cause two types of acid-base disturbance. First, the salicylates stimulate the respiratory center, which produces marked hyperventilation and respiratory alkalosis. The salicylates then cause a disturbance in metabolism, which results in increased accumulation of acids in the body and metabolic acidosis. When there is a combination of types of imbalance, treatment must be vigorous to prevent death.

combination

It is possible to have a single type of acid-base imbalance or a _____ of types of imbalance.

Effects of acidosis and alkalosis on the body

178 The major effect of acidosis is depression of the central nervous system. When the pH of the blood falls below 7, the nervous system becomes so depressed that the person is disoriented and later may be comatose. The main effect of alkalosis on the body is overexcitability of the nervous system. This occurs both in the central nervous system and in the peripheral nerves, with the peripheral nerves usually affected first. As a result of repeated stimulation by nerves, the muscles go into a state of tetany or tonic spasm. A patient with alkalosis may die from tetany of the respiratory muscles. The symptoms of central nervous system stimulation are nervousness and convulsions.

depression

a Acidosis causes _____ of the central nervous system.

stimulation

b Alkalosis causes _____ of the central and the peripheral nervous systems.

SUMMARY

Respiratory acidosis or alkalosis is the result of some disease or conditon that affects the respiratory system. In respiratory acidosis there is interference, causing increased amounts of carbon dioxide to remain in the body. This results in an increase of carbonic acid. In respiratory alkalosis there are decreased amounts of carbon dioxide in the body and consequently less carbonic acid. In respiratory acidosis the kidneys assume responsibility for correcting the imbalance by conserving base bicarbonate and excreting hydrogen ions. In respiratory alkalosis the kidneys excrete bicarbonate ions and retain hydrogen ions.

Metabolic acidosis is the result of a loss of base, and metabolic alkalosis results from an excessive intake of base. Therefore both the respiratory system and the renal system contribute to return the pH to the normal body level. In metabolic acidosis there are increased quantities of acid in relation to the available base in the intravascular fluid. Therefore the body compensates by hyperactive breathing to exhale more carbon dioxide, and the kidneys excrete more hydrogen ions. In metabolic alkalosis there is an increase of base in the intracellular fluid. Respirations become suppressed to increase the carbon dioxide and consequently the carbonic acid. The kidneys retain hydrogen ions and excrete bicarbonate ions to return the pH of the extracellular fluids to a normal level.

REVIEW

1 When carbon dioxide is retained in the intravascular fluid, the result is an increase of _____.

carbonic acid

2 An increase of carbonic acid in the intravascular fluid results in _____.

acidosis

3 When acidosis exists, the kidneys excrete _____ _____.

hydrogen ions

4 In metabolic alkalosis more base bicarbonate is available; therefore the respiratory system becomes _____ _____ and retains _____.

suppressed
carbon dioxide

5 In metabolic alkalosis the kidneys excrete _____ _____ and retain _____.

bicarbonate ions
hydrogen ions

6 The major effect of acidosis on the nervous system is _____.

depression

65

Blood gas analysis

179 In acid or base imbalance some of the effects are not very specific. Therefore the blood gas analysis is the most useful way to identify the imbalance.

The most useful test to identify an acid or base imbalance is the _____ analysis.

blood gas

180 Arterial blood is best for blood gas analysis. Arterial blood gas analysis measures pH, arterial oxygen tension (Po_2), arterial carbon dioxide tension (Pco_2), and either standard plasma bicarbonate (HCO_3^-) or carbon dioxide content. (When a gas such as carbon dioxide is dissolved in a liquid, the concentration of the gas in the liquid is directly proportional to the partial pressure. "P" stands for partial pressure.) The normal range of arterial pH is 7.35 to 7.45; the normal range of arterial Po_2 is 80 to 110 mm Hg; and the normal range of arterial Pco_2 is 35 to 46 mm Hg.

7.35 to 7.45
80 to 110
35 to 46

a The normal arterial pH is _____.
b The normal arterial Po_2 is _____.
c The normal arterial Pco_2 is _____.

181 The arterial blood gases have the same normal values in children as in adults. However, during the first month of life infants have values that are slightly lower than those of children and adults. In a newborn the pH has a normal range of 7.27 to 7.42; the normal range of arterial Po_2 is 60 to 80 mm Hg; and the normal range of Pco_2 is 30 to 40 mm Hg.

In a newborn the arterial blood gas values are (the same as? lower than? higher than?) those in a child or an adult.

lower than

182 The base component is evaluated in some laboratories by the standard bicarbonate, but in others the carbon dioxide content is used instead. The latter is a more useful test, since it measures both elements of the acid-base proportion and permits an accurate assessment of the clinical problem. The carbon dioxide content represents the sum of all forms of carbon dioxide in the blood, which includes that dissolved in the plasma (measured as P_{CO_2}), that derived from bicarbonate (HCO_3), and that derived from plasma carbonic acid (H_2CO_3). The normal carbon dioxide content is 24 to 33 mEq/L, or an average of 28 mEq/L in an adult. The normal value for standard plasma bicarbonate is 22 to 26 mEq/L in an adult.

In an infant the normal carbon dioxide content is 20 to 28 mEq/L, which is lower than that in an older child or an adult. The normal value for standard plasma bicarbonate is 22 to 26 mEq/L in an adult and slightly lower, 20 to 26 mEq/L, in an infant.

a The base component is measured by the standard bicarbonate or the carbon dioxide content. The normal average carbon dioxide content for an adult is _____ mEq/L.

28

b The base component, whether measured by the standard bicarbonate or the carbon dioxide content, in an infant is (slightly higher than? the same as? slightly lower than?) in an adult.

slightly lower than

183 In examining arterial blood gas values you should look at the pH first. The pH is the prime indicator of acidosis or alkalosis.

acidosis

a A pH of 7.24 would indicate (acidosis? alkalosis?).

alkalosis

b A pH of 7.56 would indicate (acidosis? alkalosis?).

184 You should look at the P_{CO_2} to determine the respiratory parameter. If the P_{CO_2} is increased, it indicates that more carbon dioxide is being retained. If the P_{CO_2} is decreased, it indicates that more carbon dioxide is being exhaled. A high P_{CO_2} is an indication of respiratory acidosis.

above

In respiratory acidosis the P_{CO_2} will be (above? below?) normal.

185 The next part of the arterial blood gas analysis, which will help you determine the type of acid-base imbalance, is the base component. This is the metabolic parameter. The carbon dioxide content (base) will be increased in metabolic alkalosis.

In metabolic acidosis the carbon dioxide content (base) will be (increased? decreased?).

decreased

Summary of normal blood gas analysis	
pH	7.35 to 7.45
Po_2	80 to 110 mm Hg
Pco_2	35 to 46 mm Hg
CO_2 content	24 to 33 mEq/L
Standard bicarbonate	22 to 26 mEq/L

Respiratory acidosis

186 Respiratory acidosis is the result of an increased level of carbonic acid in the extracellular fluid that is caused by an inadequate exchange of gases in the lungs, with retention of carbon dioxide. Conditions that may cause respiratory acidosis include depression of respirations by drugs or disease, foreign objects in the airway, and trapping of air in portions of the lung (as occurs with emphysema and pneumonia).

Any condition in which there is retention of carbon dioxide may cause ______________________.

respiratory acidosis

187 Signs we need to recognize in assessment that may indicate respiratory acidosis include distressed respirations, anxiety, disorientation, confusion, and body weakness.

a One sign of respiratory acidosis is (easy? distressed?) respirations.

distressed

b A person who has respiratory acidosis is likely to be (oriented? disoriented?).

disoriented

188 If the respiratory acidosis is severe, the person may become unconscious or may develop ventricular fibrillation.

It is possible for a person in severe respiratory acidosis to develop an arrhythmia of the heart such as ______________________.

ventricular fibrillation

189 According to laboratory findings, in respiratory acidosis that is uncompensated the pH will be low and the partial pressure of carbon dioxide (Pco_2) will be high. The carbonic acid concentration cannot be measured directly in the hospital laboratory. However, the carbonic acid concentration is proportional to the partial pressure of the carbon dioxide, and this can be measured. Since carbon dioxide is retained, the P_{CO_2} will be high. The normal range of P_{CO_2} is 35 to 46 mm Hg. The average P_{CO_2} in arterial blood is 40 mm Hg, whereas the average P_{CO_2} in venous blood is 46 mm Hg.

a The normal range for pH in extracellular fluid is

7.35 to 7.45 _____.

35 to 46 **b** The normal range of P_{CO_2} is from _____ mm Hg.

low **c** In respiratory acidosis the pH will be (high? low?).

high **d** The P_{CO_2} will be (high? low?).

190 As the buffer systems and kidneys compensate for the acidosis, the pH will return to normal. The P_{CO_2} may return to more nearly normal but likely will remain elevated if the cause of the respiratory acidosis is not corrected. The pH can return to normal even though carbon dioxide is retained in the body because the kidneys conserve bicarbonate ions and excrete hydrogen ions to achieve balance.

As the body compensates for the acidosis, the pH will

return to normal likely (remain low? return to normal? remain high?).

191 Normal breathing must be restored as much as possible. Treatment is aimed at the cause of the inadequate exhalation of carbon dioxide. Drugs that further depress respiration should not be given.

Deep respirations at regular intervals will aid in re-

breathing storing normal _____.

192 The elevated P_{CO_2} must be reduced gradually. Intermittent mechanical ventilation is sometimes used to help reduce the P_{CO_2}.

Mechanical ventilation may be used in treating re-

P_{CO_2} spiratory acidosis to reduce the elevated _____.

193 Nursing interventions include maintaining a patent airway, aspiration of excessive respiratory secretions, and artificial respiration if necessary. Medications and parenteral fluids may be necessary to restore balance. In extreme cases parenteral fluids that contain lactate or bicarbonate may be ordered by the physician.

Adequate ventilation is the main treatment for

respiratory acidosis _____.

194 Oxygen may be ordered when anoxia is present. However, in a person with chronic retention of carbon dioxide (e.g., as occurs in emphysema), oxygen may endanger the patient. Normally, as the level of carbon dioxide increases, the medulla and chemoreceptors stimulate respirations. In a person with a chronic elevation of carbon dioxide, the respiratory center becomes insensitive to the level of carbon dioxide. Respirations are stimulated instead by a decreased oxygen level.

increased
a Normally respirations are stimulated by (increased? decreased?) carbon dioxide.

oxygen
b In a person with chronic retention of carbon dioxide, respirations are stimulated by low levels of _____.

195 If oxygen is administered to a person with a chronically elevated P_{CO_2}, observe the patient closely because respirations could be depressed to the point of cessation.

Oxygen should be used cautiously in the person with

P_{CO_2}
chronic elevation of _____.

Respiratory alkalosis

196 Respiratory alkalosis results from a deficit in carbonic acid that is caused by hyperventilation. It is a common type of acid-base imbalance. Respiratory alkalosis may result from intracranial lesions or high temperature.

Any condition in which there is a loss of carbon dioxide can cause

respiratory alkalosis
ide can cause _____.

197 One of the earliest indications of respiratory alkalosis is a tingling sensation in the fingers and toes. This is due to the stimulation of the nervous system. Other symptoms that may occur if the alkalosis is severe include palpitation, perspiration, tetany, and heart arrhythmias.

The earliest indication of respiratory alkalosis is a

tingling sensation
_____ in the fingers and toes.

198 In respiratory alkalosis the laboratory findings show the pH to be higher than normal and the P_{CO_2} to be low. This is just the reverse of the laboratory findings in respiratory acidosis.

high **a** In respiratory alkalosis the pH will be _____.

low **b** In respiratory alkalosis the P_{CO_2} will be _____.

199 As the body compensates for the alkalosis, the kidneys will conserve hydrogen ions.

bicarbonate If the kidneys retain more hydrogen ions, they will excrete more _____ ions.

200 The treatment of respiratory alkalosis is aimed at increasing the level of carbon dioxide. This can be done by having the patient rebreathe a mixture of his own carbon dioxide and oxygen from a large paper bag or by giving inhalations of 5% carbon dioxide at intervals.

carbon dioxide Treatment of respiratory alkalosis should increase the level of _____.

Metabolic acidosis

201 A patient with mild metabolic acidosis may have no symptoms. The acidosis is due to a decrease in the alkali reserve. It may be caused by a loss of bicarbonate from the gastrointestinal tract or the kidneys or from excessive production of acid. The nurse will assess for general malaise or weakness and a dull headache. Nausea, vomiting, and abdominal pain may also be present.

Early signs of metabolic acidosis include general malaise and headache that may be accompanied by the following gastrointestinal symptoms:

nausea **a** _____

vomiting **b** _____

abdominal pain **c** _____

202 As the acidosis increases in severity, the person may become confused and finally unconscious.

In acidosis the central nervous system is depressed.

confusion; unconsciousness Therefore _____ and then _____ may occur.

203 The laboratory findings include a low pH and a low standard bicarbonate. The normal value for standard plasma bicarbonate ranges between 22 and 26 mEq/L. Normal carbon dioxide content is 24 to 33 mEq/L, or an average of 28 mEq/L.

below

a In metabolic acidosis the pH is (above? below?) normal.

below

b If the standard bicarbonate is measured in metabolic acidosis, it will be (above? below?) normal.

content

c Instead of measuring standard bicarbonate, the laboratory may report the carbon dioxide _____.

28

d The average normal value for carbon dioxide content is _____ mEq/L.

204 A decreased pH will stimulate the respiratory center to exhale more carbon dioxide and thus reduce the carbonic acid. Therefore another sign in metabolic acidosis is deep and rapid respirations. The laboratory values will be different in uncompensated and compensated metabolic acidosis. In uncompensated metabolic acidosis the pH will be low, the P_{CO_2} will be normal, and carbon dioxide content will be low (as is standard bicarbonate).

low

In uncompensated metabolic acidosis the standard bicarbonate will be low and the carbon dioxide content will be (high? low?).

205 When compensation occurs, the pH rises slightly but may remain below normal. The P_{CO_2} falls because of hyperventilation. If the kidneys can conserve bicarbonate ions, the standard bicarbonate will rise toward normal (as will the carbon dioxide content).

below

In partially compensated metabolic acidosis the pH, standard bicarbonate, and carbon dioxide content will return to more nearly normal but will remain slightly (below? above?) normal.

206 Treatment is aimed at correcting the cause of the metabolic acidosis. In severe acidosis the physician will order fluids to be given to correct the base bicarbonate deficit. Alkalinizing solutions such as sodium bicarbonate or lactate-containing solutions may be given parenterally.

Treatment with parenteral fluids include solutions to

base bicarbonate   correct the deficit of _____.

Metabolic alkalosis

207 Metabolic alkalosis is the result of excessive base bicarbonate and may occur because excessive base was taken orally or given parenterally. It also may occur when hydrochloric acid is lost from the body by vomiting or through suction.

Remember: the effect of alkalosis on the central ner-

stimulation   vous system is _____.

208 Therefore the symptoms we can expect because of central nervous system stimulation include paresthesias (abnormal sensations such as numbness and prickling), restlessness, confusion, and tetany.

In the laboratory findings we would expect the pH to

above   be (above? below?) normal.

209 The standard bicarbonate content and carbon dioxide content in metabolic alkalosis are the opposite of those found in metabolic acidosis.

In metabolic alkalosis the standard bicarbonate and

above   carbon dioxide content will be (above? below?) normal.

210 The aim of treatment is to correct the problem that produced the metabolic alkalosis. Then treatment is directed at replacing lost acid in the form of fluid or medication containing chloride. In metabolic alkalosis caused by vomiting, usually there will also be a deficiency of potassium, in which case potassium chloride may be ordered by the physician.

A chloride-containing solution or medication would

metabolic alkalosis   likely be used in treating _____.

General nursing responsibilities

211 We have considered the signs, laboratory results, and treatment for the four types of acid-base imbalance. It should be evident that overtreating one type of imbalance may upset the balance in the opposite direction. We

73

shall now consider general nursing responsibilites in acid-base imbalance. The nurse must make pertinent assessments. These will include the state of consciousness, restlessness, type of respirations, skin color, and vital signs. In observing the patient's state of consciousness, the nurse will need to know whether he is oriented, alert, or drowsy but rouses easily or whether he responds only to pain.

consciousness

The nurse must assess the state of _____ of the patient.

212 In addition to the patient's state of consciousness, the nurse should observe whether the patient is quiet or restless and the character of his respirations.

The nurse must assess whether the patient is restless and what is characteristic of the patient's

respirations

_____.

213 So far we have considered observation for state of consciousness, restlessness, and character of respirations. The nurse should also observe the skin for color changes and whether it is moist or dry.

color

In assessing the skin, the nurse looks for changes in _____ and determines whether the skin is moist or dry.

214 The nurse should assess the state of consciousness, restlessness, type of respirations, skin color and moisture, and vital signs. In taking the pulse rate, the nurse should look especially for irregularities in rhythm.

irregularities

In taking the pulse, the nurse should be alert to _____ in rhythm.

215 In addition to making pertinent assessments the nurse must protect the patient from injury. Since a person with acid-base imbalance may have either depression or stimulation of the central nervous system, the nurse must protect such a patient from injury during unconsciousness or convulsions. Protection of the patient from injury is an important nursing responsibility.

unconsciousness

a In acidosis the patient will have depression of the central nervous system that could cause _____.

convulsions

b In alkalosis the nervous system is stimulated, and the patient may have _____.

216 The nurse should make **pertinent** assessments, protect the patient from injury, and provide both physiological and psychological comfort.

comfort

The nurse should provide physiological and psychological _____.

217 Another important nursing responsibility for patients with acid-base imbalance is accurate recording of intake and output. The type and volume of fluids taken as well as lost will be important in determining treatment. A record of intake and output is especially important in infants and elderly persons.

intake

output

An accurate record of both _____ and _____ is important for the patient with either acid or base imbalance.

218 The nurse should make **pertinent** assessments, protect the patient from injury, provide comfort, and record intake and output. The **nurse** must also be able to perform the necessary therapeutic procedures as indicated. This might include catheterization and hourly analysis, venipuncture for diagnostic tests and parenteral fluids, and other nursing procedures.

hourly analysis

The nurse may need to **perform** therapeutic procedures, such as catheterization, for the purpose of _____.

SUMMARY

Acid-base imbalance caused by a disturbance in the level of carbonic acid is called *respiratory* acidosis or alkalosis. The laboratory criteria useful in determining the degree of imbalance are the pH and P_{CO_2}. In respiratory acidosis the pH will be low and the P_{CO_2} will be high. Treatment is aimed at relieving the cause of retention of carbon dioxide and then giving base or alkali to restore balance. In respiratory alkalosis the pH will be high and the P_{CO_2} will be low. Treatment is aimed at increasing the retention of carbon dioxide.

In *metabolic* acidosis and alkalosis the problem is the level of base bicarbonate or alkali. In metabolic acidosis the level of base bicarbonate is less than normal and therefore the acid side of the balance is high. The laboratory findings include a low pH and standard bicarbonate and carbon dioxide content. Treatment is aimed at correcting the cause of the imbalance and replacing base. In metabolic alkalosis there is an excess of base, which is indicated by a high pH and standard bicarbonate and carbon dioxide content. Treatment is directed toward supplying acid.

In both types of acidosis, respiratory and metabolic, the central nervous system is depressed. The nurse must be alert for symptoms such as disorientation, confusion, lethargy, and malaise. If the degree of acidosis increases in severity, the patient may become unconscious. In respiratory acidosis, respirations may be distressed. In metabolic acidosis there may be gastrointestinal symptoms of nausea, vomiting, and abdominal pain.

In both types of alkalosis, the central nervous system is stimulated. Therefore the nurse should be alert to signs of paresthesia, restlessness, confusion, and tetany. If the degree of alkalosis increases in severity, convulsions may occur.

The nurse must assess and report signs and symptoms that may indicate an acid or base imbalance. The patient must be protected from injury. The nurse should also provide comfort and keep a record of intake and output.

REVIEW

1 Distressed respirations are likely to occur in and may produce _____.

respiratory alkalosis

2 A patient who has respiratory acidosis is likely to be (oriented? disoriented?).

disoriented

3 In a patient with chronic retention of carbon dioxide, respirations will be stimulated by low levels of _____.

oxygen

4 In respiratory alkalosis the P_{CO_2} will be _____.

5 Nausea, vomiting, and abdominal pain sometimes

metabolic acidosis

occur in _____.

6 In uncompensated metabolic acidosis the standard bi-

low

carbonate and carbon dioxide content are _____.

7 The nurse should make pertinent observations, protect the patient from injury, provide comfort, perform thera-

intake

peutic procedures, and record _____

output

and _____.

CASE STUDIES

Jamie Smith

1 Jamie Smith is 6 weeks old, and his mother reports that he has begun to vomit after each feeding. She is breast-feeding him, and he nurses hungrily. Earlier he would occasionally "spit up" some after a feeding, but not like he has in the past few days. This morning it was projectile. Yet Jamie seems to be hungry. The vomitus smells sour and is the color of milk. You notice that his respirations are shallow and are slower than expected.

His blood gas report is as follows:

pH is 7.49
Po_2 is 88 mm Hg
Pco_2 is 35 mm Hg
CO_2 content is 37 mEq/L

alkalosis

a Jamie's pH of 7.49 tells you he has (acidosis? alkalosis?).

normal

b His Pco_2 of 35 is _____.

high

c His CO_2 content of 37 is _____.

metabolic alkalosis

d It is likely that Jamie has _____.

2 In infants the most common cause of metabolic alkalosis is loss of hydrochloric acid (HCl) through vomiting secondary to hypertrophic pyloric stenosis.

Jamie has developed metabolic alkalosis because of

hydrochloric acid

loss of _____.

3 It is important for Jamie to have his alkalosis corrected before he has treatment for his hypertrophic pyloric stenosis. He needs to have the chloride replaced, as well as other electrolytes that may be low. It is also likely that he needs to have fluid volume replaced.

Jamie should have treatment for his metabolic alkalosis (before? after?) treatment for his hypertrophic pyloric stenosis.

before

Laura Hart

1 Laura Hart, 18 years old, has come to the physician's office with symptoms of polyuria (frequent urination), polydipsia (excessive thirst), tiredness, and muscular weakness. She is breathing deeply and rapidly.

Her laboratory findings include glucose and acetone in her urine and a blood sugar level of 560 mg/100 ml. Her plasma pH is 7.02; her Pco_2 is 19 mm Hg.; and her CO_2 content is 5 mEq/L.

acidosis

a Ms. Hart's pH of 7.02 indicates that she has (acidosis? alkalosis?).

low

b Her Pco_2 of 19 is (low? normal? high?).

very low

c Her CO_2 content of 5 is (very low? slightly low? normal? high?).

2 With her deep and rapid respirations, Ms. Hart will lose more _____.

carbon dioxide

Her rapid respirations are a defense mechanism to get rid of more CO_2 so there will be less (carbonic acid? bicarbonate?).

carbonic acid

3 Since Ms. Hart's respiratory system can assist in compensating for her acidosis, her pH is not as low as it would be without that mechanism. Her acidosis is (metabolic? respiratory?).

metabolic

4 Ms. Hart's treatment needs to be aimed at lowering her blood sugar level, along with adding fluids to correct the base bicarbonate deficit. Since her base bicarbonate level is lower than normal, the acid side of the balance is (high? low?).

high

5 A possible nursing diagnosis for Ms. Hart could be

anxiety/fear related to diagnosis of diabetes and potential complications of diabetes. Fear can likely be alleviated by giving Ms. Hart (accurate? no?) information about her disease.

accurate

Robert Jones

1 Robert Jones is a 50-year-old man who has been admitted to the hospital in a state of coma. The history indicates that he has had chronic obstructive lung disease for the past 6 years, and during the past 2 weeks he became increasingly weak and disoriented.

Mr. Jones' blood gas report is as follows:

pH is 6.8

Po_2 is 55 mm Hg

Pco_2 is 95 mm Hg

CO_2 content is 35 mEq/L

acidosis

very high

respiratory acidosis

a Mr. Jones' pH of 6.8 tells you he has _____.

b His Pco_2 of 95 is (low? normal? high? very high?).

c Mr. Jones has _____.

2 Mr. Jones' pH of 6.8 is at the lower limit that is compatible with life. Unless he has active treatment, his acidosis will result in _____.

death

3 Mr. Jones also has hypoxia, with a Po_2 of 55, which needs to be treated along with his respiratory acidosis. Mr. Jones has a (serious? slight?) acid-base imbalance.

serious

4 A possible nursing diagnosis for Mr. Jones could be activity intolerance related to insufficient oxygenation secondary to chronic impaired gas exchange. The signs and symptoms that support this nursing diagnosis include _____ respirations and _____.

distressed

weakness

Mary Baker

1 Mary Baker, age 8, has been practicing for a swimming race for several weeks. She is a strong swimmer, but she is afraid she will not win this one. As she is getting

79

ready to begin the race, she is breathing rapidly and deeply so she can go as far as possible under water. Suddenly she sits down and says her lips and hands are numb. You notice that her hands are in carpal spasm. She says she feels as though she will faint.

a You know that with deep and rapid breathing, more

carbon dioxide

_____ is exhaled and lost from the body.

b With less carbon dioxide available, there will be a deficit of

carbonic acid

_____.

respiratory alkalosis

c The acid-base imbalance Mary has is _____

_____.

2 The treatment for respiratory alkalosis is to increase the level of carbon dioxide. One way you could do this would be to have Mary rebreathe _____

her carbon dioxide and oxygen mixture

_____ by holding a paper bag over her mouth and nose.

PART 3 Fluid volume imbalance

INTRODUCTION

Illness is usually accompanied by some disturbance of body fluids, either locally or systemically. The nurse must know what the various body fluid disturbances are, how they develop, and what characterizes them. You have completed the program that presents the normal distribution and constituents of body fluids, as well as the controls for maintaining fluid and electrolyte balance. As a nurse you share with the physician the responsibility for making observations that will serve as a basis for decisions regarding the fluid and electrolyte status of the patient. The nurse is available to make assessments not only of the patient's output, but also of his intake, as well as symptoms and signs relative to his fluid needs.

Fluid volume imbalance is more likely to occur and to be severe in infants and in the elderly than in children or younger adults. The greater need of infants for fluid and their larger surface area relative to their size contribute to their potential for fluid imbalance. In addition, infants have a higher metabolic rate with greater heat production and insensible fluid loss, along with a greater need for fluid excretion. Kidney function is immature at birth, with a limited capacity to concentrate or dilute urine. In the elderly there is homeostatic fragility along with decreased total body water. With increasing age there is a reduced sensation of thirst and declining urinary concentrating ability, which may be due to poor renal response to the antidiuretic hormone (ADH) and may be related to the decreased number of nephrons in the kidney. Therefore assessing for fluid imbalance in infants and the elderly becomes especially important.

219 You may recall that the chief sources of fluid in health are

ingestion of liquids   **a** _____

water in solids   **b** _____

metabolism (water of oxidation)   **c** _____

_____

220 Normally fluid losses occur through the gas-

kidneys   trointestinal tract, the lungs, the skin, and the _____.

FLUID VOLUME DEFICIT

221 A deficit in the fluid volume may occur for two reasons. It may be simply the result of an inadequate intake, or it may result from the fact that the loss (output) is increased over the intake. Water alone may be lost, but more likely electrolytes will be lost as well. The loss of one (water or electrolytes) may be greater than the loss of the other.

Water deficit may be due to

inadequate intake   **a** _____

excessive output   **b** _____

222 Whenever the loss of water from the body exceeds the intake, water is extracted from the extracellular fluid compartment. The result is that the remaining extracellular fluid becomes hypertonic in relation to the intracellular fluid.[3]

According to the law of osmosis, water can be ex-

out of   pected to move (out of? into?) the cell.

223 This results in cellular _____

dehydration or crenation   _____.

82

224 Since the extracellular fluid becomes hypertonic, the osmotic pressure is increased. The increase in osmotic pressure in the extracellular fluid stimulates the sensation of thirst. Elderly persons are likely to have an impaired sense of thirst and therefore may not drink enough fluid.

a When water is available and the person is able to ingest and absorb it, fluid volume deficit can be corrected by _____.

drinking water

b Elderly persons may not drink enough fluid because of an impaired sense of _____.

thirst

225 When the osmotic pressure of the cells becomes relatively less than that of the extracellular water, the posterior pituitary gland secretes more ADH.[8] When no ADH is secreted, the volume of urine excreted is five to ten times normal. Then the extracellular fluids become more concentrated. At the other extreme, when large quantities of ADH are secreted, excessive amounts of water are resorbed and the volume of urine may become less than one third the normal volume. Extracellular fluids then become more dilute.

In a fluid volume deficit, as a result of the decreased blood volume flowing through the kidneys and the increased secretion of ADH, normally functioning kidneys will excrete (more? less?) urine.

less

226 When there is a fluid volume deficit, the volume of extracellular water is decreased. This causes the adrenal glands to secrete aldosterone, which causes a retention of sodium that further increases the hypertonicity of the extracellular fluid.

Therefore cellular dehydration is (increased? decreased?).

increased

Laboratory findings

227 Because of a deficit of volume, the hematocrit (the proportion of erythrocytes to blood plasma) will be elevated. A normal hematocrit is 40% to 45% for women

Table 3. Hematocrit in children

	Age
Newborn	53% to 65%
Infant	30% to 40%
Child	31% to 43%

From Behrman RE and Vaughn VC: Nelson textbook of pediatrics, ed 13, Philadelphia, 1987, WB Saunders.

and 45% to 50% for men. A normal hematocrit for infants is 30% to 40%, and it is 31% to 43% for children.

higher

a The normal hematocrit for a newborn is (higher? lower?) than any other age group (see Table 3).

higher

b In a person with a deficit of fluid volume, the hematocrit will be (higher? lower?) than normal for his age group.

increased

228 Since the volume of fluid is decreased, the ratio of sodium and other electrolytes in the plasma will be (increased? decreased?).

229 The healthy kidneys adapt by excreting a small volume of concentrated urine. The normal specific gravity of urine is 1.010 to 1.025. In adults with adequate kidney function, an output of less than 500 to 800 ml in 24 hours is indicative of inadequate water intake.

Both infants and the elderly have a decreased ability to concentrate urine. Therefore they are more likely to develop a deficit of fluid volume.

Which of the following test results would indicate fluid volume deficit? (See page 13 for normal electrolyte values.)

_____ **a** Serum sodium 140 mEq

√ _____ **b** Hematocrit 55% in a 3-year-old

√ _____ **c** Specific gravity of urine 1.040

_____ **d** Serum chloride 103 mEq

Who of the following are most likely to be unable to concentrate urine?

√ _____ **a** 3-month-old Jill

_____ **b** 10-year-old Angie

_____ **c** 40-year-old Mr. Brown

√ _____ **d** 92-year-old Mrs. Graham

Signs and symptoms

230 In assessing a patient, the nurse will look for signs and symptoms of fluid volume deficit. Thirst is the earliest symptom of water deficit and occurs when the water loss is equal to about 2% of body weight.[8] This would be about 1400 ml in a person weighing 70 kg. As extracellular fluid is lost, the osmotic pressure of the remaining fluid is increased and water moves from the cells into the extracellular compartment. Therefore the intracellular fluid volume is decreased. Apparently, the hypothalamus is sensitive to the decreased intracellular fluid volume and produces the sensation of thirst. Patients who are apathetic, confused, or very ill are likely to develop a water deficit. The sense of thirst may be impaired in infants, in persons with cerebral arteriosclerosis, in persons with cerebral injury, and in the elderly. Patients with an elevated temperature lose excessive amounts of water from the lungs. In patients with a tracheostomy, an accelerated pulmonary water loss is likely because the dead air fraction of the tidal volume is reduced. An excessive loss of water may occur in patients with burns. The nurse should anticipate the possible fluid volume deficit and see that adequate amounts of water are given in a palatable form.

The following are likely to need additional fluid intake:

apathetic and confused patients

a _____
_____

patients with elevated temperature

b _____
_____

tracheostomy patients

c _____

burn patients

d _____

infants

e _____

patients with cerebral injury

f _____

elderly patients

g _____

231 In an alert, competent person the earliest symptom

thirst

of a fluid volume deficit is _____.

232 A fluid volume deficit is also likely to occur when swallowing is difficult or when the patient is comatose.

85

Persons with diabetes insipidus cannot concentrate water because of a lack of ADH. Persons with intrinsic kidney disease may have an inability to conserve water. The nurse should be alert to other signs and symptoms when thirst is not indicated by the patient. When the water deficit is approximately 6% of body weight, the skin and mucous membranes may provide signs to indicate the fluid volume status.[8] In a person weighing 70 kg, this would be a deficit of about 4200 ml. Dry, cracked mucous membranes are indicative of an inadequate fluid intake. However, a dry and fissured tongue may also occur in a person who is a mouth breather or is receiving oxygen by mask. The skin may be flushed, and perspiration decreased. There is little saliva, and the urine output is decreased to less than 500 ml in 24 hours in an adult. Thirst is a symptom of fluid volume deficit in alert persons. The nurse should also be aware of signs of fluid volume deficit.

Which of the following signs may indicate fluid deficit?

_____ **a** Moist, clean mucous membranes
√   _____ **b** Urine output of 400 ml in 24 hours in an adult
_____ **c** Cool, moist skin
√   _____ **d** Dry, fissured tongue

233 If, in addition to the signs just mentioned, the patient has marked physical weakness and confusion or delirium, the water deficit is likely to be 7% to 14% of body weight. In a patient weighing 70 kg, this would be approximately 5000 to 10,000 ml.[8] The blood pressure will also decrease.

Signs of severe water deficit include

weakness   **a** _____

delirium or confusion   **b** _____

decreased blood pressure   **c** _____

234 In infants a fluid volume deficit is a very common problem that is often caused by gastroenteritis. Since an infant has a relatively greater body surface area, large quantities of fluid can be lost through the skin. Remember (frame 87) that infants ingest and excrete a greater amount of fluid per kilogram of body weight than do older children or adults.

greater

a An infant has a relatively (smaller? greater?) body surface area than an adult.

skin

b Infants can lose a significant quantity of fluid through the _____.

235 Dehydration (fluid volume deficit) is one of the most common body fluid disturbances in infants and children. Whenever the output of fluid exceeds the intake, dehydration occurs.

The most common body fluid disturbance in infants

dehydration

is _____.

236 There are three types of dehydration: isotonic, hypotonic, and hypertonic. In isotonic dehydration there is a loss of fluid and electrolytes in approximately balanced proportion. Most of the loss is sustained from the extracellular compartment.

In isotonic dehydration there is a loss of both electro-

fluid

lytes and _____.

237 Isotonic dehydration is the most common type of dehydration. Another type is hypotonic dehydration. Hypotonic dehydration means that the electrolyte deficit is greater than the fluid deficit. Since the extracellular fluid is hypotonic, there is movement of extracellular fluid into the intracellular space. Therefore the extracellular fluid volume becomes even less. The physical signs and symptoms tend to be more severe with hypotonic dehydration.

In hypotonic dehydration the deficit of electrolytes is

greater

(less? greater?) than the deficit of fluid.

238 The third type of dehydration is hypertonic. As you can guess, hypertonic dehydration means that the deficit of fluid is greater than the deficit of electrolytes. Since fluid will then shift out of the intracellular space and into the extracellular space, the physical signs and symptoms of fluid volume deficit are not as apparent, but neurological disturbances become evident.

Table 4. Physical signs of dehydration

	Isotonic (loss of water and salt)	Hypotonic (loss of salt in excess of water)	Hypertonic (loss of water in excess of salt)
Skin			
Color	Gray	Gray	Gray
Temperature	Cold	Cold	Cold or hot
Turgor	Poor	Very poor	Fair
Feel	Dry	Clammy	Thickened
Mucous membranes	Dry	Slightly moist	Parched
Tearing and salivation	Absent	Absent	Absent
Eyeball	Sunken and soft	Sunken and soft	Sunken
Fontanel	Sunken	Sunken	Sunken
Body temperature	Subnormal or elevated	Abnormal	Subnormal or elevated
Pulse	Rapid	Very rapid	Moderately rapid
Respirations	Rapid	Rapid	Rapid
Behavior	Irritable to lethargic	Lethargic to comatose; convulsions	Marked lethargy with extreme hyperirritability on stimulation

From Whaley LF and Wong DL: Nursing care of infants and children, ed 4, St. Louis, 1991, Mosby–Year Book, Inc.

into   **a** In hypertonic dehydration fluid shifts (into? out of?) the extracellular compartment.

less   **b** In hypertonic dehydration the physical signs and symptoms of fluid volume deficit are (more? less?) apparent than in hypotonic dehydration.

239 Since infants and small children are unable to describe their symptoms, the nurse must be observant to detect changes (see Table 4). In isotonic and hypotonic dehydration, skin turgor is lost. However, in hypertonic dehydration the skin will feel firm.

lost   In isotonic dehydration skin turgor is (lost? firm?).

240 The mucous membranes become dry with isotonic dehydration. The eyeballs appear sunken and soft. The fontanel becomes sunken or depressed. The infant's pulse and respirations are rapid.

Which of the following may indicate an isotonic dehydration?

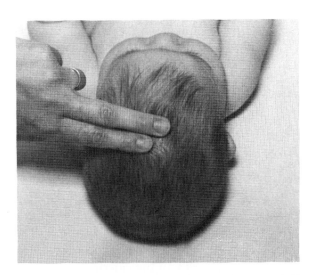

Palpating anterior fontanel. (From Whaley LF and Wong DL: Nursing care of infants and children, *ed. 4, St. Louis, 1991, Mosby–Year Book.)*

_____ **a** Moist, mucous membranes
_____ **b** Soft, sunken eyeballs
_____ **c** Depressed fontanel
_____ **d** Slow pulse and respirations

241 Another significant change is a decrease in weight from the pre-illness weight. The urine output will also decrease, along with an increase in specific gravity. Any other sign or symptom must also be recorded and reported.

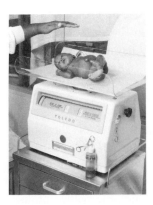

From Perry AG and Potter PA: Clinical nursing skills and techniques, *ed. 2, St. Louis, 1991, Mosby–Year Book.*

a With a fluid volume deficit, the infant's weight will

decrease

_____.

b The specific gravity of the urine will _____.

increase

242 Dehydration is the most common cause of fluid and electrolyte disturbance in the elderly. This is partially due to the decrease in total body water and to the reduced thirst, along with the reduction in urinary concentrating ability that occurs with increasing age.

decreased

a One cause for dehydration in the elderly is (increased? decreased?) thirst.

less

b With increasing age, the kidneys become (less? more?) able to concentrate urine.

243 In the elderly, tissue turgor decreases with the loss of subcutaneous fat, which results in wrinkling of the skin. This should not be interpreted as a sign of dehydration.

is not

Wrinkled skin in the elderly (is? is not?) always a sign of dehydration.

244 For most situations of fluid volume deficit the nurse monitors the patient to detect signs and/or symptoms and collaborates with the physician for treatment. Therefore it is a collaborative or interdependent problem rather than a nursing diagnosis. In a situation of decreased sense of thirst the nursing diagnosis could be fluid volume deficit related to inadequate oral intake secondary to decreased sensation of thirst. The nurse would then plan to provide oral intake for the patient. Since the nurse can order and provide treatment, a nursing diagnosis is appropriate.

When the nurse can order and provide treatment, a

is

nursing diagnosis (is? is not?) appropriate.

Overhydration

245 Another cause of fluid volume deficit is giving large amounts of fluid to the patient too rapidly. We could suppose that giving water when there is a fluid volume deficit would correct the imbalance. However, this is true only within limits. If a very large volume of fluid is given intravenously or if the person drinks an excessively large volume of water, the urine output may be greatly increased.

Although not a common cause, a deficit of fluid
volume   _____ can be produced by giving *excessive* amounts of water.

SUMMARY

Whenever the loss of water from the body exceeds the intake, water is extracted from the extracellular fluid compartment. Since the extracellular fluid becomes hypertonic, the osmotic pressure is increased and thirst results. The nurse must be alert to conditions in which water deficit could exist and observe and report any signs and/or symptoms. Marked physical weakness and confusion are signs of severe water deficit.

REVIEW

1 When the volume of fluid is decreased, the concentration of sodium and other electrolytes in the plasma
increased   will be _____.

2 When there is a deficit in the fluid volume, the hema-
elevated   tocrit will be _____.

3 The following are likely to need additional fluid:

apathetic, confused, and   **a** _____
very ill patients   _____

patients with elevated   **b** _____
temperature   _____

tracheostomy patients   **c** _____

burn patients   **d** _____

infants   **e** _____

patients with cerebral injury **f** _____

4 Signs of fluid deficit include the following:

dry, cracked mucous   **a** _____
membranes   _____

flushed skin   **b** _____

decreased urine output   **c** _____

5 Signs of fluid deficit in an infant include the following:

eyeballs sunken and soft
a _____

fontanel sunken or depressed
b _____

rapid pulse and respirations
c _____

weight loss
d _____

Fluid requirements

246 Average fluid requirements for adults

Intake

Ingested liquids	1500 ml
Water in foods	700 ml
Water formed in metabolism	200 ml
TOTAL	2400 ml

Output

Kidneys	
Urine	1400 ml
Lungs	
Water in expired air	350 ml
Skin	
Diffusion	350 ml
Perspiration	100 ml
Intestine	
Feces	200 ml
TOTAL	2400 ml

In a person with normally functioning kidneys, the volume of urine output is a good clue to the adequacy of the fluid intake.

The average volume of urine per 24 hours for an adult is approximately _____ ml.

1400

247 An average adult requires approximately 1500 to 2000 ml of water per day. If a person has a marked elevation of temperature, an additional 500 to 1500 ml of water is necessary daily.[8]

Therefore a person with an elevated temperature will need from _____ ml of water over a 24-hour period.

2000 to 3500

248 If a person is perspiring moderately, an additional 500 ml of water is needed. If the perspiration is profuse, another 1000 ml of water is necessary.

Table 5. Pediatric fluid intake

Weight	Kilogram body weight formula	Example weight	Example total fluid per 24 hr
Newborn	60-100 ml/kg	3 kg	180-300 ml
0-10 kg	100 ml/kg	8 kg	800 ml
11-20 kg	1000 ml for first 10 kg, plus 50 ml/kg over 10 kg	15 kg	1250 ml
21-30 kg	1500 ml for first 20 kg, plus 25 ml/kg over 20 kg	25 kg	1625 ml

In part from Hazinski MF: Nursing care of the critically ill child, St. Louis, 1991, Mosby–Year Book, Inc.

Pediatric urine output

Newborn	50-300 ml/24 hr
Infant	350-500 ml/24 hr
Child	500-700 ml/24 hr
Adolescent	700-1400 ml/24 hr

From Behrman RE and Vaughn VC: Nelson textbook of pediatrics, ed 13, Philadelphia, 1987, WB Saunders.

3000 to 4500

A person who has a temperature of 104° F and is perspiring profusely may need _____ ml of fluid over a 24-hour period.

249 Other causes for increased loss of fluid include vomiting, diarrhea, gastrointestinal drainage, burn exudate, internal pooling, wound exudate, etc.

A fluid volume deficit can be the result of an inadequate intake or an _____.

excessive or increased loss

250 Average fluid requirements for children are given in Table 5, and urine output is indicated in the box.

In a child the average output is approximately half that of an adult.

The average volume of urine per 24 hours for a child is approximately 500 to _____ ml.

700

251 The average newborn infant requires 60 to 100 ml/kg of fluid over a 24-hour period, which would be approximately 240 ml/24 hr for a 3 kg (7 pound) infant.

240

A 3 kg newborn infant would require approximately _____ ml of fluid over a 24-hour period.

252 Fluid needs in children are based on their weight.

A 3-year-old child weighing 15 kg (33 pounds) would require approximately _____ ml of fluid over a 24-hour period.

1250

253 If an infant or child has an elevated temperature and is perspiring, a proportionate increase will need to be added to his maintenance fluid requirements.

A child with an elevated temperature and who is perspiring will need (an increased? a decreased?) amount of fluid.

an increased

254 In the elderly there is a decrease in the total amount of body fluid; therefore their need for liquid intake is slightly less than that of younger adults. However, since aging kidneys are less able to concentrate urine, their output will remain high and will require an equal amount of intake.

Even though the total body water is less in the elderly, their intake and output (do? do not?) change significantly from younger adults.

do not

Treatment

255 Pure or distilled water can be given only orally. For many persons a water deficit can be prevented by providing adequate amounts of water in a clean, palatable form. The most satisfactory way is for the patient to drink from a glass or cup while in the sitting position. For alert patients this may be all that is necessary to increase fluid intake. Some patients, especially infants, children, and elderly persons, may require assistance. For patients who must remain supine, their heads should be turned to the side if possible. Some patients should be given an explanation of how much fluid intake is desirable and why.

The most satisfactory way to provide fluid intake for children and adults is_____

_____.

drinking from a glass while sitting up

94

Fluids by infusion

256 Water can be given orally, except when fluids by mouth are contraindicated.

We established earlier (frame 60) that distilled water cannot be infused because it is hypotonic and cells would _____ and _____.

swell; burst

257 The physician determines which fluids will be given parenterally. However, fluids given intravenously should be isotonic or only slightly hypotonic or hypertonic.

When fluids are given intravenously, they should be (hypotonic? isotonic? hypertonic?) to the extracellular fluid.

isotonic

258 One example of an isotonic solution that could be given intravenously is dextrose 5% in water.

Dextrose 5% in water is a/an (hypotonic? isotonic? hypertonic?) solution.

isotonic

259 The potential danger to the patient is increased when fluids are given intravenously because fluids go immediately into the systemic circulation. Although the physician is responsible for the prescription of the amount, character, and route of administration of the patient's intake, the nurse is usually responsible for the administration of the fluids. Therefore the nurse must know how to give fluids in a safe and effective manner. The nurse also must be sure that the patient gets the correct solution, the proper amount, and at the rate prescribed. The nurse must also see that sterility of the solution and the equipment is maintained.

The nurse is responsible for (prescription? administration?) of fluids.

administration

260 In giving any medication, the nurse checks that the right drug in the proper dose, time, and method of administration is given to the right patient.

To give intravenous fluids safely and effectively, the nurse should identify the patient and see that he gets the right _____, in the proper _____ at the _____ prescribed.

solution; amount
rate

261 All patients should be observed regularly when fluids are given parenterally. The nurse should not rely on the patient to check the rate of infusion. The patient has neither the training nor the experience to know what to look for. The patient's energy should be conserved for recovery. Observation is especially important in patients whose homeostatic mechanisms are inadequate or defective. Patients with limited renal and/or cardiac reserve are in danger of pulmonary edema or congestive heart failure. Very young, as well as older patients, are less able to tolerate large volumes of fluid given rapidly. The nurse is responsible for the safe administration of fluids.

renal
cardiac

Pulmonary edema or congestive heart failure is more likely to occur in patients with limited _____ and/or _____ reserve.

262 The nurse should be alert to symptoms that indicate congestive heart failure. If the patient becomes short of breath or has dyspnea (difficult breathing), the flow rate should be decreased and the physician notified. An increase in the respiratory rate, the occurrence of coughing, or the development of cyanosis suggests an overloading of the patient's circulation, with movement of fluid into the alveoli of the lungs.

Pulmonary edema and congestive heart failure are likely to be accompanied by the following symptoms:

shortness of breath
dyspnea
increased respiratory rate
coughing
cyanosis

a _____
b _____
c _____
d _____
e _____

263 The rate of administration of intravenous fluids depends on the need for fluids and the nature of the fluid. The physician will prescribe exactly how fast the fluid should be given intravenously. The rate of flow will affect the safety and the state of comfort of the patient. Fluids given over a 12- to 24-hour period contribute more to the patient's comfort and to fluid and electrolyte balance than do fluids administered over a shorter period. The rate of flow affects the value of the fluids to the patient.

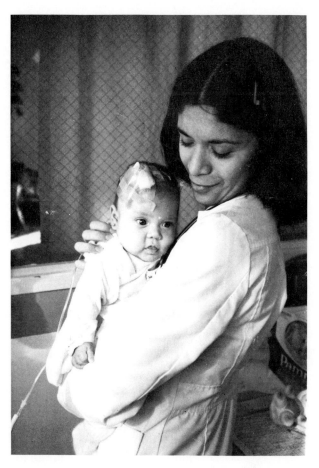

Intravenous infusion does not prevent infant from being picked up and cuddled. (From Whaley LF and Wong DL: Nursing care of infants and children, ed. 4, St. Louis, 1991, Mosby–Year Book.)

12 to 24

Fluids given over a period of (4 to 12? 12 to 24?) hours will be safest and most effective.

264 The rate of administration varies with the condition of the patient and the nature of the fluid. However, the patient must be observed frequently. Shortness of breath or dyspnea may indicate that the rate is too rapid. The nurse must be alert to the patient's urinary output in relation to the fluid intake and observe and report signs of too rapid a rate of administration.

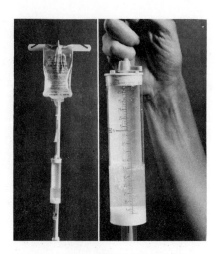

From Perry AG and Potter PA: Clinical nursing skills and techniques, *ed. 2, St. Louis, 1991, Mosby–Year Book.*

decreased

A patient who is receiving intravenous fluids and who becomes short of breath or dyspneic should have the rate of fluid flow (increased? left the same? decreased?).

265 When fluids are being given intravenously to infants and children, accurate intake is essential. The rate of administration of the fluids must be kept constant. Therefore some type of volume control device is used with infants and children (see the illustration on this page). Even a very small error could cause serious problems. Rates in children generally vary from 5 to 80 ml/hr depending on the size of the child, whereas the rate for an adolescent or adult could be 80 to 150 ml/hr.

The rate for intravenous fluids in a child varies from

5

_____ to 80 ml/hr.

Calculating the rate of flow

266 The rate of administration of fluids intravenously can be calculated when we know the drop size for the administration set we are using. The size of the drops varies in the different parenteral administration sets. We should know how many drops are needed to give 1 ml (1 cc) with the administration set being used. The variation in size of drops with different commercial administration sets is as follows:

Approximate no. of drops to deliver 1 ml

Company	Regular set	Pediatric set
Abbott and McGraw	15	60
Baxter and Travenol	10	50
Cutter and IVAC	20	60

When we divide the number of drops per minute by the number of drops per milliliter that our administration set gives, we find the number of milliliters per minute. To find how many milliliters are being given per hour, we then multiply by 60 (60 minutes = 1 hour). If we were using an Abbott set, which requires 15 drops for each milliliter, we would use the drops per minute, divide by 15, and then multiply by 60. We may arrive at the same figure if we use a shortcut that Goldberger calls the drop factor[8]: we divide 60 (the minutes in 1 hour) by 15 (the number of drops per milliliter) to get 4. In this example, 4 is our drop factor; to find the milliliters per hour, we multiply the drops per minute by the drop factor.

a If the administration set requires 15 drops for 1 ml of fluid and the fluid is flowing at 25 drops/min, the patient will be receiving _____/hr.

25 × 4 = 100 ml

b If we use a drop factor of 4 and the rate is 35 drops/min, the patient will receive _____/hr.

35 × 4 = 140 ml

c If we use an administration set requiring 10 drops for 1 ml, our drop factor will be _____.

60 ÷ 10 = 6

267 Now suppose we are to give 1000 ml of fluid in 8 hours. We need to know first how many milliliters per hour are desired.

a 1000 ml ÷ 8 = _____ ml/hr.

125

The drops per minute necessary are found by dividing the milliliters per hour by the drop factor.

b If the administration set requires 15 drops/ml, the drop factor will be _____.

60 ÷ 15 = 4

c The number of drops per minute necessary to give 1000 ml of fluid in 8 hours is _____.

125 ml ÷ 4 = 31

268 We have an order to give 4000 ml of fluid in 24 hours.

If the administration set requires 15 drops/ml, how shall we calculate the drops per minute required to give 4000 ml in 24 hours? (Round off fractions to nearest whole number.)

$4000 \div 24 = 167$ ml/hr

$60 \div 15 = 4$ (drop factor)

$167 \div 4 = 42$ drops/min

a _____

b _____

c _____

269 To check our answer, we multiply the drops per minute by the drop factor to get the milliliters per hour.

168

a $42 \times 4 =$ _____.

We then multiply the milliliters per hour times the number of hours.

4032

b $168 \times 24 =$ _____.

Mechanical factors affecting flow rate

270 A change in needle position may alter the flow rate. If the bevel of the needle is against the wall of the vein, the rate will be slower than normal. A change in the height of the bottle of fluid above the needle site will alter the rate. The greater the height of the bottle above the needle site, the faster the rate of flow.

If we raise the bottle of fluid higher, the rate of flow will (increase? not change? decrease?).

increase

271 If we keep the bottle of fluid the same height above the floor and raise the level of the patient's bed, the flow rate will _____.

decrease

272 The patency of the needle will alter the flow rate. A change in position of the limb may affect the rate.

Mechanical factors that influence the flow rate of intravenous fluids include the following:

change in needle position

patency of needle

change in position of limb

change in height of bottle above patient

a _____

b _____

c _____

d _____

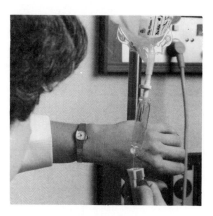

Rate of infusion should be checked by watch. (From Perry AG and Potter PA: Clinical nursing skills and techniques, *ed. 2, St. Louis, 1991, Mosby–Year Book.)*

Adjusting rate of flow

273 Since the intravenous infusion is most effective when spaced over a long period of time, the infusion rate must remain nearly constant (except in emergency situations). However, after the rate is adjusted, continuous supervision is required to see that it does not change because of mechanical factors. In adults the rate should be checked at least every hour. In infants and children the rate should be counted and recorded every 15 minutes.

a In children the rate of intravenous infusion should be counted every _____ minutes.

15

b In adults the rate of intravenous infusion should be counted every _____.

hour

274 If a liter of fluid is to be given over a period of 8 to 12 hours, the bottle or plastic bag should be labeled as to how many milliliters per hour are to be administered ("1000 ml 5% dextrose in saline to run for 8 hours"). In this way the nurse can tell quite accurately whether the rate is still adjusted correctly. A piece of adhesive or masking tape can be used to indicate the milliliters to be given per hour and where the level of fluid should be each hour. Although this method works best on a glass

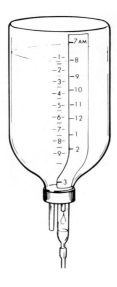

or rigid container, an approximate level can be indicated on any container.

a If 1000 ml is started at 7 AM and is to be given over a period of 8 hours, _____ milliliters should be given by 11 AM.

500

b By 1 PM, _____ should be given.

750 ml

275 Hypertonic and hypotonic solutions should be given at a slower rate than isotonic solutions. (See box on p. 103 for examples of isotonic, hypertonic, and hypotonic solutions.) One of the best guides to a safe rate of flow is the reaction of the patient. Therefore the nurse must observe signs and symptoms carefully.

Symptoms of pulmonary edema include the following:

shortness of breath **a** _____

dyspnea **b** _____

coughing **c** _____

cyanosis **d** _____

increased respiratory rate **e** _____

276 If these symptoms occur, the nurse should

slow the rate of infusion **a** _____

notify the physician **b** _____

(Refer to frame 262, if necessary.)

```
Intravenous fluids

Isotonic solutions

5% dextrose in water
Sodium chloride solution (0.9%) (normal saline)

Hypertonic solutions

10% dextrose in normal saline
3% sodium chloride
5% sodium chloride

Hypotonic solutions

One-half hypotonic saline (0.45%)
5% dextrose in 0.45% saline

Isotonic fluids with multiple electrolytes

Plasma-Lyte
Isolyte E
Lactated Ringer's solution (Hartmann's)
Ringer's solution

Hypotonic fluids with multiple electrolytes

Isolyte R
Normosol-M
Plasma-Lyte
Ionosol B
```

slowed

277 If the patient becomes short of breath, the rate of infusion should be (slowed? increased?).

278 The maximum rate for administration of glucose to normal adults without producing glycosuria is approximately 0.5 g per kilogram of body weight per hour (0.5 g/kg/hr).[3] At this rate it would take approximately 1½ hours to administer 1000 ml of 5% dextrose in water or saline solution to a patient weighing 70 kg (154 pounds), or twice as long for 1000 ml of 10% dextrose. The exact rate at which fluids are to be infused should be determined by the physician. A safe method of determining the rate of fluid administration is to divide the volume of fluid to be given by 24 hours.

24-hour

The safest method of fluid administration is to give the fluids over a _____ period.

279 If the rate of infusion exceeds the suggested maximum rate, the body is unable to metabolize the glucose. Therefore it is excreted in the urine. This further increases the output of fluid, since more fluid is required in which to dilute the glucose for excretion.

The maximum rate at which the body can metabolize glucose is _____ g per kilogram of body weight per hour.

0.5

SUMMARY

The volume of urine output serves as a good indication of the adequacy of fluid intake in anyone with normally functioning kidneys. When there is a fluid volume deficit, fluids can be given orally or parenterally. The nurse is responsible for the administration of fluids and must be alert to the dangers when fluids are given parenterally. Dyspnea, increased respiratory rate, coughing, and cyanosis are symptoms that indicate an overload of the patient's circulatory system. Since the patient will benefit more from an intravenous infusion if it is spaced over a longer period of time, the nurse must know how to calculate and adjust the rate of flow.

REVIEW

1 At the morning report you are told that Mr. Green, a 53-year-old man who has had a cerebral vascular accident, had a urine output of 400 ml for the past 24 hours.

24-hour intake

a Next you should find out his _____.

b You would need to collect additional data, but a possible nursing diagnosis for Mr. Green might be fluid volume deficit related to unknown cause.

24 hour output

c The only evidence you have in this situation is his _____.

2 Mrs. Cole, a 90-year-old woman who was admitted yesterday, is receiving fluids intravenously. You note that her respiratory rate is increasing and she is beginning to cough frequently.

slow the rate of infusion

a Your first action should be to _____
_____.

b Based on the data you have, a possible nursing diagnosis for Mrs. Cole could be fluid volume excess related to excessive intake and/or decreased output. The signs and symptoms supporting this diagnosis are _____ and _____.

increased respiratory rate; cough

3 Mr. Berry, who has had a cerebral vascular accident and is unable to swallow, is to receive 3000 ml of fluid intravenously. He will get the most benefit from the fluids if they are (spaced over a 24-hour period? run very rapidly?).

spaced over a 24-hour period

4 Rosa, 7 months, was admitted to the hospital because of dehydration. The physician has ordered the intravenous infusion to run at 50 ml/hr.

15 minutes
a You should check the rate of flow every _____.

deficit
b A nursing diagnosis for Rosa could use the category of fluid volume (deficit? excess?). We do not have data to indicate the cause, therefore we cannot write a nursing diagnosis unless we say it is related to an unknown cause, or wait until we have more data.

FLUID VOLUME EXCESS

280 Just as it is possible to develop a fluid volume deficit, so it is possible to have an excess of extracellular fluid volume. Fluid volume excess is not likely to occur unless the renal mechanisms fail. The cause of fluid excess may be diseased kidneys, excessive secretion of ADH, or decreased blood flow through the kidneys. Decreased blood flow through the kidneys is likely to occur in elderly persons. The cause of fluid excess is the same in children as in adults. As in fluid volume deficit, the electrolytes are out of balance along with fluid volume excess. When there is an increase in the extracellular fluid volume, the osmotic pressure is reduced because there is a decrease in the number of particles per unit of water.[3] As a consequence, fluid moves from the extracellular compartment into the cell.

swell
Therefore the cells (swell? shrink?).

281 Normally, when a person takes an excess of water and water moves into the cells, this causes the osmoreceptors to respond and the posterior pituitary decreases the secretion of ADH. As a result, the excess fluid is excreted by the kidneys. However, if a patient has an excessive secretion of ADH, then the water will be retained. Therefore more fluid will move into the cells.

less Normally, excess fluid in the cells causes the posterior pituitary to secrete (more? less?) ADH.

282 When the secretion of ADH is decreased, the urinary output is (increased? decreased?).

increased

283 There are several reasons why a patient may have excessive secretion of ADH. Excessive secretion of ADH can occur as a result of fear, pain, or acute infections. It can also occur as a result of most anesthetics or analgesics such as morphine or meperidine hydrochloride (Demerol). Any acute stress (such as trauma or a major operation) may stimulate excessive secretion of ADH. Postoperatively the excessive secretion of ADH may last 12 to 36 hours or longer.[3] Oxytocin has antidiuretic properties and may cause volume excess if injected along with an infusion of dextrose and water.[8] Accurate measurement of intake, output, and the patient's weight is important after any acute stress.

increase **a** The effect of stress on the secretion of ADH is to (increase? decrease?) secretion.

decreased **b** This results in (increased? decreased?) excretion of fluid.

284 An excessive secretion of ADH is likely to occur in which of the following situations?

√ _____ **a** Twenty-four hours after cholecystectomy

√ _____ **b** A patient who had a coronary occlusion yesterday and continues to have severe pain

√ _____ **c** A patient who is receiving meperidine, 100 mg every 3 hours, for pain from a ureteral calculus

_____ **d** A patient who had a fractured femur pinned 10 days ago

√ _____ **e** A postpartum patient who was hemorrhaging and was given oxytocin in an intravenous solution of 5% dextrose in water

285 Some persons with cerebral lesions or lung cancer may have excessive secretion of ADH.

As the secretion of ADH increases, the excretion of

decreases — urine _____.

286 Whenever there is a low renal blood flow and the kidneys are unable to excrete urine, fluid volume excess is likely to occur. In persons with adrenal cortical insufficiency or acute renal insufficiency, excessive retention of water occurs because the kidneys do not excrete water. In severe congestive heart failure or cirrhosis of the liver the renal blood flow is low. Therefore the kidneys are unable to excrete normal amounts of fluid.

An excess of fluid volume is likely to occur in a person with severe congestive heart failure because of the

decreased — decreased renal blood flow, which results in (increased? unchanged? decreased?) urinary output.

287 Water excess can occur if large volumes of water are given rectally because the water comes in contact with the absorbing surface of the colon. Patients who have lost sodium are likely to develop water excess because the osmotic pressure of the extracellular fluid is lower than that of the cells.

Giving large amounts of water rectally may result in

excess — fluid volume (excess? deficit?).

Signs and symptoms

288 Fluid volume excess can be prevented if the nurse carefully observes and reports the patient's total fluid intake and output. Changes in the patient's weight can provide data that, when added to other facts, will indicate the fluid volume status. For each pound of weight gained, about 1 pint of fluid (500 ml) is retained. An acute weight gain, in excess of 5% of body weight, may indicate fluid excess.[5]

a In a person weighing 150 pounds, this would be a

7½ — weight gain of _____ pounds.

b An acute gain in weight may be indicative of fluid

excess — volume (excess? deficit?).

c When there is a fluid volume deficit, the extracellular

107

hypertonic   fluid becomes (hypotonic? isotonic? hypertonic?).

d When there is a fluid volume excess, the extracellu-
hypotonic   lar fluid becomes ＿＿＿＿＿＿＿.

e When the extracellular fluid is hypotonic, fluid will
into   move (into? out of?) the cell.

289 As fluid moves into the cells, the cells swell. The symptoms that patients have in fluid volume excess are the result of disturbed cerebral function. In severe fluid volume excess the patient develops unusual behavior, loss of attention, confusion, and aphasia. This may be followed by convulsions, coma, and death.[3]

    In fluid volume excess, symptoms due to disturbed cerebral function include

unusual behavior   **a** ＿＿＿＿＿＿＿＿＿＿＿＿＿＿＿＿＿＿＿＿

loss of attention   **b** ＿＿＿＿＿＿＿＿＿＿＿＿＿＿＿＿＿＿＿＿

confusion   **c** ＿＿＿＿＿＿＿＿＿＿＿＿＿＿＿＿＿＿＿＿

aphasia   **d** ＿＿＿＿＿＿＿＿＿＿＿＿＿＿＿＿＿＿＿＿

290 In fluid volume excess the skin is warm and moist and may be flushed. The cardiovascular system remains normal as long as the excess fluid volume remains in the interstitial spaces or does not become too great. Edema may occur in dependent parts of the body or in the lungs, especially if the person has congestive heart failure.

    Which of the following may indicate fluid volume excess?

√   ＿＿ **a** Warm moist skin

    ＿＿ **b** Cool dry skin

√   ＿＿ **c** Mental confusion

    ＿＿ **d** Loss of weight

√   ＿＿ **e** Convulsions

291 In a person with congestive heart failure who has a fluid volume excess, the likely symptoms include edema of dependent body parts and lungs. Symptoms of edema or fluid in the lungs are the same as those discussed in fluid volume deficit when fluid is given too rapidly and pulmonary edema results. Also, the blood pressure may rise.

    Symptoms of pulmonary edema include the following:

shortness of breath	**a** _____
dyspnea	**b** _____
coughing	**c** _____
cyanosis	**d** _____
increased respiratory rate	**e** _____

decreased

292 The hemoglobin and hematocrit levels are (increased? decreased?) because of the fluid volume excess.

293 The mean corpuscular volume (MCV) of the erythrocytes is increased because the osmotic pressure in the extracellular fluid is lower than that of the cells.

drawn into

Therefore water is (drawn into? pushed out of?) the cells.

294 If a postoperative patient develops unusual behavior, has a convulsive seizure, experiences hemiplegia, or becomes comatose, fluid volume excess should be suspected. The water-excess syndrome that follows surgery or trauma is usually self-limited. However, if the person has a convulsion or hemiplegia or becomes comatose, death may follow even though active treatment is given.

The nurse must keep an accurate record of fluid intake, output, and weight of patients in the first few days after surgery or trauma, for these persons are suscepti-

excess

ble to fluid volume _____.

serious

295 Convulsions or hemiplegia caused by fluid volume excess are indicative of (self-limited? serious?) fluid volume excess.

Treatment

296 Fluid volume excess may be treated by limiting the fluid intake. How much the fluid intake is restricted depends on the condition of the patient. The physician will determine the amount of fluids the patient may take in. If the patient has renal failure, the fluid intake may be limited to 300 to 500 ml in 24 hours.[3] If the patient has had a convulsion or is experiencing hemiple-

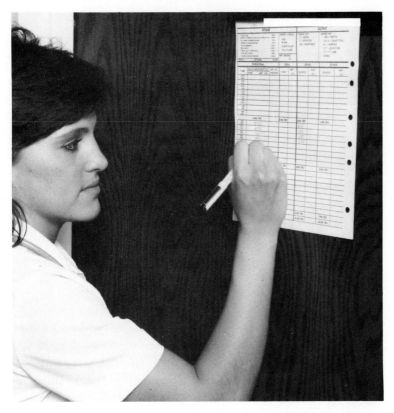

From Perry AG and Potter PA: Clinical nursing skills and techniques, *ed. 2, St. Louis, 1991, Mosby–Year Book.*

gia, fluids must be withheld and a hypertonic saline solution should be given.[8] In infants and children a proportionate amount of fluids should be withheld. The nurse should work with the dietary department and space the amount of fluid the patient may have over 24 hours.

In an adult, in acute renal failure the fluid intake may be limited to _____ ml in 24 hours.

300 to 500

297 If the fluid volume excess is serious, the fluid intake may be (restricted? stopped?).

stopped

298 Any acute stress may stimulate an excessive secretion of ADH, which can lead to fluid volume (excess? deficit?).

excess

299 This can be corrected before the excess becomes serious if the nurse daily collects the following data in susceptible persons:

intake **a** _____

output **b** _____

weight **c** _____

SUMMARY

Normally, when excess fluid moves into cells, the secretion of ADH is decreased; therefore the urine output is increased. However, any acute stress may stimulate an excessive secretion of ADH, which results in decreased excretion of fluid. In fluid volume excess, symptoms caused by disturbed cerebral function include confusion, loss of attention, unusual behavior, and aphasia. These may be followed by convulsions, coma, and death. The nurse must carefully observe patients likely to develop fluid volume excess and keep records of intake, output, and weight. In this way the excess fluid volume may be corrected before it becomes serious.

REVIEW

1 Mr. Short weighed 171 pounds yesterday. Today his weight is 180 pounds. After determining that this is his actual weight today, the nurse should be aware that the

fluid volume excess   gain may represent _____.

2 The nurse should look for symptoms due to fluid volume excess. Symptoms of disturbed cerebral function include the following:

unusual behavior **a** _____

loss of attention **b** _____

confusion **c** _____

aphasia **d** _____

warm and moist   **3** In fluid volume excess the skin will be _____.

excess   **4** A nursing diagnosis could be fluid volume _____ related to unknown cause, since more data is not available.

5 The signs or symptoms Mr. Short has that are given

weight gain

here and support this category are _____.

6 The first step in treating fluid volume excess is to

restrict

_____ fluid intake.

FLUID VOLUME SHIFTS

300 Fluids may shift from the intravascular compartments into the interstitial space. In some clinical disorders, depletion of the extracellular fluid develops because large quantities of fluid are held in an interstitial area, which makes them inaccessible to the body. This is called "third spacing," and the fluid is usually essentially invisible.

The term "third spacing" refers to fluids that are

not available

(available? not available?) for use by the body.

301 This shift of fluid into "third space" may be localized to a single area or organ, or it can spread throughout the body. For example, a person with ascites will have large quantities of fluid in the abdomen. A person who has had abdominal surgery may have significant quantities of fluid that are not available for use by the body. The reasons why fluids may shift into "third space" includes lowered plasma proteins, increased capillary permeability, or lymphatic blockage. These changes in the movement of fluids may be secondary to trauma, inflammation, or disease. It is a major factor in the fluid balance of persons who have had abdominal surgery.

The factors that allow fluids to move from the intravascular compartment into "third space" include

decreased

a (decreased? increased?) plasma proteins

increased

b (decreased? increased?) capillary permeability

lymphatic

c _____ blockage

302 The first phase of "third spacing" is loss. Depending on the cause, it is likely to last for 48 to 72 hours. During this time the symptoms will be those of a fluid volume deficit.

In the first phase of "third spacing" you should expect symptoms of fluid volume (excess? deficit?).

deficit

303 During this phase, fluids shift from the vascular to the interstitial spaces. The shift in fluids occurs because of increased capillary permeability in areas of inflammation and trauma. The increased capillary permeability allows plasma proteins to leak into the interstitial space. In some situations lymphatic blockage may allow fluid to remain in the interstitial spaces. When fluids shift into "third space" even though intravenous fluids are being given, the fluid does not stay in the intravascular compartment and the patient becomes hypovolemic. The person has a decreased blood volume.

When fluids shift into "third space," the blood volume or intravascular fluid volume decreases. This is called _____.

hypovolemia

304 The clinical signs you should watch for with hypovolemia include a decreased blood pressure and an increased heart rate.

decrease

a In hypovolemia the blood pressure will (increase? decrease?).

increase

b The heart rate will (increase? decrease?).

305 You will expect to find an increase in heart rate and a decrease in blood pressure when hypovolemia occurs. Also, a person with hypovolemia will have a low central venous pressure and a decreased urine output.

low

a In hypovolemia the central venous pressure will be (high? normal? low?).

decrease

b The urine output will (increase? decrease?).

306 The second phase of "third spacing" is resorption. After the inflammation subsides, the fluid in the tissue spaces begins to be resorbed. Therefore intravascular volume will increase. Usually this shift occurs gradually and fluid overload does not occur unless extra fluid is given at this time.

The second phase of "third spacing" is resorption; fluid moves into the _____ compartment.

intravascular

307 During the resorption phase, nursing observations and actions should be the same as those in fluid volume excess. The information the nurse should collect daily in susceptible persons is

intake   **a** _____

output   **b** _____

weight   **c** _____

SUMMARY

Following trauma, inflammation, or some diseases, fluid may shift from the intravascular compartment into the interstitial compartment and is not accessible to the body. This is called "third spacing." The first phase of "third spacing" is loss, and it may last for 48 to 72 hours. During this time the symptoms are those of fluid volume deficit. The second phase of "third spacing" is resorption. Usually this shift of fluids back into the intravascular space is gradual. Nursing care is aimed at observations and actions to prevent severe fluid volume deficit during the first phase and to prevent fluid volume excess during the resorption phase. The nurse must be sure to keep accurate records of intake, output, and weight. An accurate intake and output is especially important for infants and for elderly persons.

REVIEW

1 When "third spacing" occurs during the first phase, the shift of fluid is (out of? into?) the intravascular compartment.

out of

2 During the first 48 to 72 hours following trauma or inflammation, the symptoms are those of fluid volume _____.

deficit

3 The second phase of "third spacing" usually involves the movement of fluids into the _____ space.

intravascular

4 While caring for infants or elderly persons with "third spacing," the nurse should keep careful records of _____, _____, and _____.

intake; output; weight

CASE STUDIES

Lisa Davis

1 Lisa Davis, a 4-month-old infant, has been admitted to the hospital with a history of vomiting and diarrhea for 5 days. She is dehydrated and has a rectal temperature of 104° F. Her skin is dry, and her respirations are rapid and shallow, with a rate of 68/min. Her apical heart rate is 164 beats/min. Her fontanel is depressed. An intravenous infusion has been started in a scalp vein. Lisa's vomiting and frequent loose stools continue.

decreased

a You would expect her weight to be (increased? decreased?) from her pre-illness weight.

increased

b You would expect her serum sodium level to be (increased? decreased?) from the normal.

2 Lisa has a convulsion, and her respirations drop to 4/min. She has an endotracheal tube inserted and is put on a ventilator.

severe

Her fluid volume deficit is (mild? severe?).

3 An appropriate nursing diagnosis for Lisa would be fluid volume deficit related to excessive loss of fluid

T 104; dry skin; respirations 68; fontanel depressed; heart rate 164

as evidenced by _____, _____, _____, _____, and _____.

Since the nurse will collaborate with the physician in treating Lisa, this is an interdependent or collaborative problem.

James Wentzel

1 Mr. James Wentzel, age 82, has been admitted to the hospital for possible surgery to correct a urinary tract obstruction. He has been unable to void for the past 12 hours and has had urgency and frequency for several weeks.

a If Mr. Wentzel has signs of water intoxication, you would expect his skin to be _____ and

cool; moist

_____.

increased

b You would expect his weight to have (increased? decreased?).

c If Mr. Wentzel has water intoxication and his extracellular fluid is hypotonic, you would expect him to be

confused

(alert? confused?).

115

d The nurse will continue to assess Mr. Wentzel for changes in his signs and symptoms and will collaborate with his _____.

physician

John Winn

1 John Winn is a 22-year-old man who was hospitalized after a gunshot wound in his abdomen. Two days ago he had surgery to repair a perforated colon and duodenum. He has a nasogastric tube in place, and it is functioning well. This morning he complains of more abdominal discomfort. You notice that his abdomen is distended. When you take his vital signs, his heart rate has gone from 86 up to 116 beats/min and his blood pressure has dropped from 130/84 to 100/68.

You should think about the possibility that Mr. Winn may have a shift of fluid _____,

into the interstitial space

also called _____.

"third spacing"

2 You would expect that his urine output has _____.

decreased

3 Your nursing action will be to report the change to the physician.

The signs and symptoms you will report include abdominal distention and discomfort, as well as his _____ and _____.

heart rate; blood pressure

116

PART 4 Electrolyte imbalance

INTRODUCTION

Each electrolyte has special functions in the body. Although some electrolytes play larger roles than do others, all are necessary for the maintenance of life. There are four basic physiological processes for which electrolytes are essential: (1) promotion of neuromuscular irritability, (2) maintenance of body fluid osmolality, (3) regulation of acid-base balance, and (4) distribution of body fluids between the fluid compartments.

We shall consider the special functions of sodium, potassium, magnesium, and calcium.

308 The physiological processes for which electrolytes are essential include the following:

neuromuscular irritability   **a** _____

body fluid osmolality   **b** _____

acid-base balance   **c** _____

distribution of body fluids   **d** _____

SODIUM IMBALANCE

309 Sodium is the major cation in the extracellular fluid. In fact, it represents about 90% of all the extracellular cations. Sodium ions are especially important in regulating the voltage of action potentials. Sodium is necessary for the transmission of impulses in nerve and

117

muscle fibers. For example, if there is a deficit in the sodium concentration, there will be muscle weakness. Since sodium is the most osmotically active solute in the intravascular and interstitial fluid, it is one of the main factors that determine extracellular fluid volume. Sodium is primarily found outside the cell and is osmotically active. Therefore it plays a major role in controlling the size of the cell.

a Sodium is essential for the normal transmission of

muscles; nerves

impulses in _____ and _____.

volume

b Sodium is also necessary to maintain the _____ of extracellular fluid.

310 The level of sodium in the body is controlled by multiple factors that are not completely understood. These factors include the adrenal glands, the pituitary gland, the skin, the gastrointestinal tract, arterial pressure, and compositional changes in the extracellular fluid. The combined effect is that the kidneys are influenced to resorb more or less sodium from the blood and to excrete it in the urine.[18] For example, if the level of sodium in the body goes down, the kidneys will excrete urine that is practically free of sodium. Active resorption of sodium by the kidneys takes place in the tubules. Normally almost all the sodium is resorbed and none of it is excreted. However, if the level of sodium is high, large portions of sodium can be excreted in the urine.

most

The normal kidneys usually resorb (most? little?) of the sodium that is filtered through them.

311 If the level of sodium becomes high, normal kid-

can

neys (can? cannot?) excrete the excess sodium.

312 Most of the sodium that is resorbed is associated with chloride.

Resorbed sodium is usually in the form of sodium

chloride

_____.

313 The kidneys are extremely important in regulating sodium balance, primarily through the action of aldosterone.

The hormone from the adrenal glands that is most

aldosterone

influential in regulating sodium balance is _____.

314 Normally almost all the sodium that is filtered by the kidneys is resorbed. Most of the sodium is resorbed with chloride, but some is resorbed when sodium ions are exchanged for potassium and hydrogen ions. In the absence of aldosterone, a person can become seriously depleted of sodium and chloride.

sodium   Aldosterone is an important hormone for the regulation of _____ and chloride.

315 There are several factors that affect the rate of secretion of aldosterone. Any one or a combination of these factors stimulates the secretion of aldosterone and, consequently, the level of sodium. These factors include reduced blood volume or cardiac output, decreased extracellular sodium, increased extracellular potassium, and physical stress. Renin, which is secreted by the kidneys and causes the formation of angiotensin, also may act directly on the adrenal cortex to secrete more aldosterone when the sodium concentration is low.

aldosterone   **a** Reduced blood volume and cardiac output stimulate the production of _____ .

low   **b** Aldosterone is secreted in greater amounts when the level of extracellular sodium is (high? low?).

high   **c** The secretion of aldosterone is stimulated by a (high? low?) level of extracellular potassium.

316 In the elderly the renal blood flow decreases, the cardiac output decreases, the plasma renin activity is lower, and the stress response to sodium restriction is blunted. All of these changes that occur with aging affect the rate of secretion of aldosterone. This indicates the increased vulnerability of the elderly person to a sodium imbalance.

more   The elderly are (more? less?) likely to have a sodium imbalance than are children or younger adults.

317 The regulation of sodium in the body is very closely interwoven with the regulation of fluid volume, since the fluid volume can be adjusted by regulating the level of sodium in the body.

Because of the osmolality, as the sodium content increases, the volume of fluid will (increase? decrease?).

increase

Sodium deficit

318 Vomiting, diarrhea, or gastrointestinal drainage from suction or fistulas may cause a sodium deficit, called *hyponatremia.* "Natrium" is the Latin word for sodium, and the symbol is Na. Though normally sodium and chloride are resorbed by the kidneys, sodium may be lost from the body through gastrointestinal secretions.

Loss of secretions from the gastrointestinal tract may cause (a loss? an increase?) of sodium.

a loss

319 Sodium may be lost through the skin, as in excessive sweating, burns, and cystic fibrosis.

In sweating, as well as in burns and cystic fibrosis, sodium is lost through the _____ .

skin

320 Hyponatremia may also occur when sodium is isolated within the body and is not physiologically available, as when there is an obstruction of the small bowel and large amounts of fluid containing sodium are held in the intestinal lumen. It may occur in burns when edema accumulates at the burn site or in peritonitis when extracellular fluid is held in the abdomen. The sodium in these fluids is not available for necessary functions.

Fluid containing sodium may be isolated in the body when any of the following occurs:

small bowel obstruction

a _____

burns

b _____

peritonitis

c _____

321 Another cause of hyponatremia is renal disease, especially salt-losing nephritis.

If the kidneys are unable to resorb _____, there will be hyponatremia.

sodium

322 Although both fluid and electrolytes are lost in the previously mentioned conditions causing sodium deficit, the fluid may be more readily replaced, leaving a deficit of sodium. For example, a construction worker who is perspiring from hard work is likely to drink large quantities of water. Thus his fluid volume may be restored, but the sodium loss will not be replaced unless he also increases his intake of salt (sodium chloride).

decreased

Whenever sodium is lost from the body, the fluid volume will be (increased? decreased?).

Signs and symptoms

323 The nurse will assess for signs and symptoms that vary depending on the degree of depletion of sodium and water, as well as the rapidity of the loss. If the loss is severe and occurs suddenly, the clinical picture will be of shock. If the loss is more gradual, the symptoms will include weakness, apathy, and lassitude.

deficit

Weakness, apathy, and lassitude are symptoms of sodium (deficit? excess?).

324 Muscle weakness, fatigue, headache, hypotension, and vertigo may occur with a sodium deficit. Muscle cramps may occur, especially if the fluid is replaced without the sodium, since fluid replacement intensifies the sodium loss. In the elderly these symptoms are often attributed to aging, and the hyponatremia may be missed.

cramps

Headache, vertigo, hypotension, muscle weakness, and muscle _____ may occur in sodium deficit.

325 A person with hyponatremia also may have gastrointestinal symptoms, including anorexia, nausea, and vomiting.

A person with hyponatremia may have gastrointestinal symptoms of

anorexia   **a** _____

nausea   **b** _____

vomiting   **c** _____

326 Since the level of sodium in the body also controls the extracellular fluid volume, some of the signs and symptoms of sodium deficit will parallel those of fluid volume deficit. There will be a loss of skin turgor; that is, if the skin of the arm is picked up and released, it will tend to remain stretched and folded for a half minute or more. Normally, when the skin is picked up, it returns almost immediately to its previous shape. In the elderly, skin turgor is not a useful sign of sodium deficit, since skin loses elasticity with advancing age.

turgor   In sodium deficit the skin will show loss of _____ in children and younger adults.

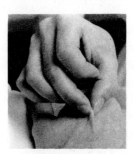

From Perry AG and Potter PA: Clinical nursing skills and techniques, ed. 2, St. Louis, 1991, Mosby–Year Book.

327 The eyeballs may be sunken and feel soft on palpation. The tongue may be wrinkled and shrunken.

In addition to a loss of skin turgor with hyponatremia, there may be changes in the eyeballs and

tongue   _____.

328 The cardiovascular signs will vary with the rate and degree of sodium loss. There may be orthostatic hypotension, which is a drop in blood pressure when the person stands and which may cause fainting.

hypotension   Hyponatremia may cause orthostatic _____.

329 There may also be tachycardia, thready peripheral pulse or loss of peripheral pulse, and collapsed neck veins.

In hyponatremia the pulse may be rapid and thready collapse   and the neck veins may _____.

330 If the hyponatremia develops slowly or is less severe, the symptoms will be less dramatic. Be alert to the possible need for sodium in the person who is fatigued, has a loss of energy, and feels faint on arising.

Hyponatremia that is not severe may cause symptoms of

fatigue   **a** _____

loss of energy   **b** _____

fainting   **c** _____

Laboratory findings

331 The hematocrit will be elevated because of hemoconcentration, yet the serum sodium will be low. The normal level of intravascular sodium is given on page 13. In hyponatremia the serum sodium will be less than 135 mEq/L. The level of sodium does not change with increasing age. The level of sodium is useful in differentiating sodium loss from water loss. In water loss a high hematocrit level is associated with a high sodium concentration.

above   **a** In hyponatremia the hematocrit will be (above? below?) normal.

below   **b** The serum sodium will be (above? below?) normal.

332 The serum level of chloride or bicarbonate will also be low. The serum potassium may be high, since some loss of sodium will cause increased retention of potassium.

low   The serum level of chloride will likely be (high? low?).

333 In sodium deficit the urinary volume will likely be low, as will the sodium and chloride concentration in the urine.

low   The urinary volume and concentration of sodium and chloride will be (high? low?).

Treatment

334 The aim of treatment is to restore balance by replacing the deficit of sodium and water. If shock exists, parenteral sodium and water will be needed. Pressor amines such as norepinephrine (Levophed) or meta-raminol (Aramine) will not be effective until some of the sodium has been replaced. A liter of isotonic saline solution (0.85%) contains 154 mEq of sodium. The amount of sodium to be replaced is calculated by the physician on the basis of the serum sodium level and the weight of the patient. The rate of flow for parenteral replacement must be carefully controlled, since too rapid replacement will increase the loss of electrolytes.

a If the hyponatremia is severe, replacement of sodium
parenteral (intravenous)   and water will be needed by the _____
route.

b The rate of flow for sodium chloride solution adminis-
controlled   tered intravenously should be (rapid? controlled?).

335 In less severe hyponatremia the sodium content of the patient's oral fluids may be increased.

orally   In some conditions sodium can be replaced _____ rather than parenterally.

336 Another aspect of treatment is to stop further loss of sodium. For example, if the patient is losing fluid from a pancreatic fistula, this fluid will have a high sodium content. Therefore isotonic saline solution should be used to replace the loss. Additional sodium chloride may be necessary.

sodium   Pancreatic drainage has a high _____ content.

SUMMARY

Sodium is the main extracellular cation. Some functions of sodium are transmission of impulses in nerve and muscle fibers, control of cell size, and maintenance of extracellular fluid volume.

Normal kidneys can selectively regulate the level of sodium in the body. Reduced blood volume, decreased cardiac output, low extracellular sodium, high extracellular potassium, and physical stress stimulate the secretion of aldosterone, which causes an increased resorption of sodium by the kidneys.

All secretions from the gastrointestinal tract contain sodium, which is normally resorbed. Therefore any abnormal loss of gastrointestinal secretions can cause a sodium deficit (hyponatremia). Sodium may also be lost through the skin or kidneys. Sudden loss of sodium may produce shock. Gradual sodium loss may be evidenced by symptoms of fatigue, loss of energy, and fainting. Other signs of hyponatremia include tachycardia and hypotension. The hematocrit will be above normal, and serum sodium will be low. Treatment is aimed at restoring balance by replacing the sodium deficit, often in the form of sodium chloride, and water deficit.

REVIEW

1 The most osmotically active extracellular cation is

sodium

_____ .

all

2 Normally almost (all? none?) of the sodium filtered by the kidney is resorbed.

increased

3 A reduced cardiac output will stimulate (increased? decreased?) secretion of aldosterone.

potassium; hydrogen

4 When sodium is resorbed because of the effect of aldosterone, more _____ and _____ ions are excreted.

sodium

5 In peritonitis, in which large amounts of extracellular fluid are held in the peritoneal cavity, there may be a _____ deficit, since this fluid is not available to the body.

increase the problem

6 In the treatment of a sodium deficit by the intravenous administration of sodium chloride, very rapid replacement may (be indicated? increase the problem?).

low

7 Ms. Bond, age 42, has been vomiting for 2 days. You would expect her serum sodium to be (high? normal? low?).

8 Which of the following signs or symptoms would you expect to find in Ms. Bond?

_____ **a** Fatigue
_____ **b** Hypertension
_____ **c** Weakness
_____ **d** Loss of skin turgor
_____ **e** Edema

√ a
√ c
√ d

9 a A possible nursing diagnosis for Ms. Bond could be fluid volume (deficit? excess?) related to low serum sodium secondary to vomiting.

Deficit

b This diagnosis is supported by the following signs or symptoms: _____, _____, and _____ .

fatigue
weakness
loss of skin turgor

Sodium excess

337 The kidneys regulate sodium excretion in a healthy person according to intake. If the kidneys fail because of hormonal or hemodynamic effects, excess sodium (hypernatremia) may develop. When this occurs, there is also fluid retention, or edema, and therefore an increase in extracellular fluid volume. For the kidneys to perform their regulatory function, an adequate blood flow must be present, as well as a normal aldosterone system. Therefore conditions in which hypernatremia may be a problem include renal failure (with sodium retention), inadequate blood circulation to the kidneys (as in congestive heart failure), cirrhosis of the liver, overproduction of aldosterone by the adrenal cortex, and use of large doses of adrenal corticoids. Since these conditions may occur in the elderly, they are likely to develop sodium excess. Elderly persons may eat more convenience-type foods, which are often high in sodium.

The kidneys must have adequate _____ and _____ to regulate the sodium level.

blood flow
aldosterone

338 Even if the kidneys do resorb increased amounts of sodium, the concentration of sodium usually will not increase significantly, since the person becomes extremely thirsty and thus drinks water, which dilutes the sodium that is resorbed. Then the problem is fluid volume excess rather than sodium excess or hypernatremia.

does not increase

Usually the concentration of sodium (increases? does not increase?) significantly, even if increased amounts of sodium are resorbed.

339 We can say, then, that hypernatremia causes increased water retention and therefore an increased extracellular fluid volume. If a person has increased resorption of sodium but is unable to take in additional fluid, the concentration of extracellular sodium will increase. Usually the concentration of extracellular sodium does not increase even with increased resorption of sodium, however, because the person drinks more fluid and therefore dilutes the retained sodium.

If a person has an increased resorption of sodium and is unable to take in additional fluid, the concentra-

increase

tion of sodium will _____ .

340 Symptoms of hypernatremia are caused by the hypertonicity of the extracellular fluids and the lack of water. Therefore the symptoms will be those of dehydration. The mucous membranes will be dry, the skin flushed, the temperature elevated, and the urine output decreased.

If there is increased resorption of sodium without an increase in fluid intake, the symptoms will be those of

dehydration

_____ .

341 Hypernatremia rarely occurs, since usually the fluid intake is increased when sodium is resorbed. The more common problem with sodium excess is an increased extracellular fluid volume that results in edema.

increase

Sodium excess is likely to cause an (increase? decrease?) in extracellular fluid volume.

342 The symptoms will depend on the location of the edema. Edema of the lungs is called *pulmonary* edema and can occur in congestive heart failure. We have considered pulmonary edema previously (frames 262 and 290).

Symptoms of pulmonary edema include the following:

shortness of breath

a _____

dyspnea	**b** _____
coughing	**c** _____
cyanosis	**d** _____
increased respiratory rate	**e** _____

343 If the edema is in the abdominal cavity, as occurs with congestive heart failure or cirrhosis of the liver, the symptoms will result from the condition causing the ascites and the pressure caused by the fluid. Edema in any tissue will interfere with the nutrition of cells because blood flow is limited to those cells.

decreased

Whenever there is edema, the cells do not have good nutrition, because blood flow is (increased? decreased?) to that part.

344 The treatment of hypernatremia accompanied by increased retention of water is aimed at the physiological mechanisms that produced the excess. For example, in the person with pulmonary edema caused by congestive heart failure, the treatment is aimed at strengthening the contractions of the heart.

sodium; water

The aim of treatment is to improve or correct the condition that caused _____ and _____ retention.

345 Another aspect of treatment is restriction of the intake of sodium. The degree of restriction will vary. For some persons, omitting salt in cooking will be an adequate restriction. For others, avoiding all salts of sodium such as sodium chloride, sodium lactate, and sodium bicarbonate may be necessary. There may be any degree of restriction between these two extremes. If salt or sodium is restricted, the nurse should be sure the patient understands the reasons for the restriction. The patient and the family must be taught how to prepare food according to the restrictions. At times the intake of water is also restricted. If water is restricted, a schedule should be worked out so that the water or fluid allowed is spaced over 24 hours.

sodium; water

In treating edema caused by retention of sodium and water, the intake of _____ and _____ may be limited.

346 Treatment may involve the use of diuretics, drugs that prevent the resorption of sodium and water.

preventing resorption

Diuretics used to treat increased retention of sodium and water act by _____ of sodium and water by the kidneys.

347 When diuretics are used, the nurse is responsible for keeping an accurate record of intake, output, and daily weight. This information is useful in avoiding overtreatment. It is possible to produce too great a loss of water and sodium as well as other electrolytes, especially potassium.

When diuretics are used, the nurse should record the following:

intake
output
daily weight

a _____
b _____
c _____

348 If the increased resorption of sodium and water is caused by the overproduction of aldosterone, an antagonist, spironolactone (Aldactone), may be used.

aldosterone

Spironolactone is an antagonist to _____.

349 The treatment of sodium and water retention will depend on the cause but may include restricting sodium and water intake and the use of diuretics.

restricting

Treatment may include _____ sodium and water intake.

SUMMARY

In a healthy person the kidneys regulate the level of sodium. Certain hormonal or hemodynamic factors may cause the kidneys to be unable to maintain this balance. The conditions in which sodium excess (hypernatremia) may be a problem include renal failure with salt retention, inadequate blood flow to the kidneys (as in congestive heart failure), cirrhosis of the liver, overproduction of aldosterone by the adrenal glands, and treatment with large doses of adrenal corticoids.

Usually, when sodium is retained, water intake and/or resorption occurs. Thus the concentration of extracellular sodium does not increase, but rather there is an increase in extracellular fluid volume. The symptoms of this increase depend on the cause and the location of the edema. Treatment may include restriction of sodium and water intake and the use of diuretics.

REVIEW

aldosterone

1 An increase in the hormone _____ will cause an increased resorption of sodium.

aldosterone

2 Inadequate blood flow to the kidneys will stimulate the production of _____, which will increase the resorption of sodium.

take in (drink)

3 When an increased amount of sodium is resorbed, the person is stimulated to _____ water.

intake

output

daily weight

4 When diuretics are used, the nurse should record

a _____

b _____

c _____

CASE STUDY
Jane Folk

1 Jane Folk, age 79, was admitted to the hospital because of vomiting and diarrhea for several days. The following morning her temperature was 105°F, her heart rate was 150 beats/min, and her respirations were 42/min. When the laboratory results were returned, her serum sodium was 153 mEq/L.

high

This serum sodium level of 153 mEq/L is (high? low?).

2 She has not been vomiting, and she has been given a limited amount of fluid intravenously. With her level of serum sodium, you would expect her to have symptoms

dehydration

of (overhydration? dehydration?).

3 Which of the following signs and symptoms would you expect her to have?

√   _____ **a** Dry, fissured tongue

√   _____ **b** Dry, warm skin

       _____ **c** Urine output of 2000/24 hr

√   _____ **d** Thirst

4 The nurse and the physician will collaborate in the medical and nursing care for Mrs. Folk. The nurse will assess, monitor, and detect signs and/or symptoms to report to the physician. When the nurse cannot order **is not** the treatment, a nursing diagnosis (is? is not?) appropriate.

POTASSIUM IMBALANCE

350 Potassium is the major cation in the intracellular fluid. However, the level of potassium inside the cell is difficult to measure, so the balance of potassium must be inferred from its extracellular or serum level. Refer to the diagrams on page 13 to compare the amount of potassium in the serum with that in the cell. Serum potassium tends to rise slightly with increasing age, especially in healthy elderly men. (See Table 7 for potassium levels in children.) The normal serum potassium level in older children and adults is 3.5 to 5 mEq/L. The serum level of potassium may or may not be an accurate index of the total body potassium. Since only 5% of total body weight is intravascular fluid and 40% is intracellu-

Table 6. Potassium levels in children

Specimen	Age	Normal value (mEq/L)
Serum/plasma	Newborn	3.7—5.0
	Infant	4.1—5.3
	Child	3.4—4.7

From Behrman, R.E., and Vaughn, V.C.: Nelson textbook of pediatrics, ed. 13, Philadelphia, 1987, W.B. Saunders Co.

lar fluid, the amount of potassium is relatively small in the intravascular fluid.

potassium

a The major cation inside the cell is _____.

3.5 to 5

b The normal level for serum potassium in older children and adults is _____ mEq/L.

351 One of the functions of potassium is to maintain the volume of fluid within the cell. We established earlier (frame 309) that sodium is important in maintaining cell size. Because sodium is the primary cation outside cells and potassium is the primary cation inside cells, both are significant in controlling the movement of fluid in and out of cells by osmosis.

potassium

a The primary cation inside cells is _____.

b The primary cation in the extracellular fluid is

sodium

_____.

c Both sodium and potassium are essential in controlling the movement of fluid in and out of cells by

osmosis

_____.

352 Potassium is important in maintaining the volume of fluid within the cell. It is also necessary for the transmission of electrochemical impulses along the membranes of nerve and muscle cells. Therefore potassium is essential in regulating neuromuscular irritability. Potassium easily diffuses through the cell membrane and thus moves positive electrical charges from inside the cell to outside the cell.

a cation

a Potassium is (a cation? an anion?).

positive

b Therefore potassium carries a (positive? negative?) electrical charge.

c Potassium is necessary for the control of electrical im-

nerve; muscle

pulses in _____ and _____ cells.

353 So far we have seen that potassium is important for the control of fluid volume within the cell and for regulating neuromuscular irritability. Another function of potassium is to control the hydrogen ion concentration. When potassium ions move out of the cell, sodium and hydrogen ions move into the cell. The usual ratio is three potassium ions for two sodium and one hydrogen ion ($3 \ K^+$ to $2 \ Na^+$ and $1 \ H^+$).

cation

sodium;
hydrogen

three; two

a When one cation moves out of the cell, another _____ moves in to take its place.

b As potassium ions move out of the cell, _____ and _____ ions move into the cell.

c This exchange of cations is usually in the ratio of _____ potassium ions for _____ sodium ions and one hydrogen ion.

354 Potassium is important in controlling intracellular fluid volume, neuromuscular irritability, and hydrogen ion concentration. The clinical signs and symptoms of potassium imbalance result primarily from altered neuromuscular irritability.

Three functions of potassium are the regulation of

intracellular fluid volume   a _____

neuromuscular irritability   b _____

H+ concentration   c _____

355 Normally potassium is ingested in the diet. Since it is present in many foods, a person who is eating a diet that is adequate in calories and protein will likely have an adequate intake of potassium. Normally a balance in the potassium level is maintained, with 80% to 90% of the potassium being excreted in the urine and the rest being eliminated in the feces and sweat.[18]

food (diet)

a Potassium normally enters the body in the form of _____.

urine

b About 80% to 90% of the potassium intake is excreted in the _____.

356 We are far from understanding how the concentration of potassium is regulated. Regardless of whether intake is low, normal, or high, there is a somewhat fixed resorption of filtered potassium in the proximal tubules that is not regulated by any known mechanism.[18] Therefore the filtered potassium is almost totally resorbed.

potassium

Resorption of filtered _____ occurs regardless of intake.

357 Although the filtered potassium is resorbed in the proximal tubules, the regulated excretion of potassium occurs in the distal tubules. The variations in excretion of potassium involve changes in potassium secretion and/or further potassium resorption.[20] This regulation of potassium excretion is related to several other processes, which include sodium resorption, hydrogen ion excretion, and aldosterone level. For potassium to be excreted, adequate amounts of sodium must be available for exchange. When there is an increase in hydrogen ion excretion, there is a decrease in potassium excretion. An increased level of aldosterone stimulates an increased excretion of potassium.

Which of the following stimulate an increased excretion of potassium?

____ **a** Sodium deficit

√ ____ **b** Decreased excretion of hydrogen ions

√ ____ **c** Increased level of aldosterone

____ **d** Acidosis

358 When body fluids become too alkaline, the kidneys preserve hydrogen ions and excrete more potassium ions in exchange. Thus with alkalosis, large amounts of potassium may be excreted in the urine.

more When alkalosis exists, (more? less?) potassium is excreted in the urine.

359 The feedback mechanism of aldosterone in regulating potassium excretion is exactly opposite that for sodium regulation. When extracellular *sodium* concentration is *low*, aldosterone secretion is increased and more sodium is resorbed. When the extracellular level of *potassium* is *high*, more aldosterone is secreted and more potassium is excreted.

excreted When the production of aldosterone is stimulated, sodium is retained in the body and potassium is ____.

Potassium deficit

360 We have considered the function of potassium and the mechanisms for its control. We shall now look at the problem of a potassium deficit. Hypopotassemia, called *hypokalemia* (from the Latin word for potassium, "kalium"), is a low serum potassium level. Remember that clinically we cannot measure the intracellular potassium. The serum potassium level may not be an accurate index of the total body potassium level.

A low serum level of potassium is called _____, or _____.

hypokalemia
hypopotassemia

361 A low serum potassium level may occur when alkalosis is present because potassium moves into the cells. In alkalosis the serum potassium level may be low even though there is not any loss of total body potassium.

In (acidosis? alkalosis?) the serum potassium level may be low even though the total body potassium level is normal.

alkalosis

362 Potassium loss causes a metabolic alkalosis, and the reverse is also true. A metabolic or respiratory alkalosis causes hypokalemia.

Alkalosis causes and can be caused by _____ .

hypokalemia

363 When potassium ions are lost from cells, sodium and hydrogen ions move into the cells to replace the potassium. Therefore the hydrogen ion concentration is decreased in the extracellular fluid and metabolic alkalosis results.

Hypokalemia will lead to metabolic (acidosis? alkalosis?).

alkalosis

364 We shall now consider some of the causes of hypokalemia. In general, hypokalemia is caused by either a decreased intake of potassium or an increased loss of potassium.

Hypokalemia may be caused by (increased? decreased?) intake and/or by _____ loss.

decreased
increased

365 Since normal kidneys continue to excrete some potassium, the body must replace it. Normally the intake of potassium is adequate in food and fluids. In a patient who is unable to eat a normal diet, potassium must be given by medication orally or via intravenous fluids. If a patient is given large amounts of intravenous fluids without potassium, hypopotassemia will result.

In a patient who is unable to eat a normal or ade-

will

quate diet, supplements of potassium (will? will not?) be necessary.

366 Even with an adequate intake of potassium, hypokalemia may occur if there is excessive loss of potassium. One way potassium may be lost is through the gastrointestinal tract. Vomiting, gastric suction, intestinal fistulas, or diarrhea can cause a severe potassium loss.

A serious depletion of potassium can occur when gastrointestinal secretions are lost through

vomiting   **a** _____

gastric suction   **b** _____

intestinal fistulas **c** _____

diarrhea   **d** _____

367 Hypokalemia may occur through loss of fluids from the gastrointestinal tract. Loss of potassium may also occur through the urinary tract in several conditions. A high sodium intake or excessive administration of bicarbonate or other alkaline substances will stimulate the urinary loss of potassium.

More potassium will be lost in the urine if the intake

high   of sodium is (high? low?).

368 Another cause of hypokalemia is certain diseases of the kidneys. Hypokalemia may occur in renal tubular acidosis, in potassium-losing nephritis, and when the patient has had a ureteroenterostomy.

Hypokalemia may occur in certain kidney diseases

increased   because of (increased? decreased?) excretion of potassium.

369 Potassium can be lost in the urine as a result of treatment with diuretics. The thiazides and furosemide (Lasix) cause loss of potassium and are more likely to cause hypokalemia in the elderly than in younger adults. While potassium-sparing diuretics (such as triamterene) are more likely to cause *hyper*kalemia in elderly persons than in younger adults, hypokalemia is likely to occur whenever certain diuretics are used, even though they may be necessary in sodium and fluid volume excess.

Use of furosemide or thiazide diuretics may result in (hyper-? hypo-?)kalemia.

hypo-

370 Use of adrenal cortical steroid hormones will increase the excretion of potassium. Earlier (frames 357 and 359) we learned that increased levels of aldosterone will stimulate the excretion of potassium. Therefore overproduction of adrenal cortical hormones or prolonged treatment with steroid drugs will cause loss of potassium.

An increase in adrenal cortical steroid hormones will cause (increased? decreased?) excretion of potassium.

increased

371 We have seen that hypokalemia may be caused by inadequate intake or by increased loss of potassium.

Potassium loss may occur through the gastrointestinal tract with vomiting, gastric suction, intestinal fistulas, or _____ .

diarrhea

372 Increased amounts of potassium may be lost through the urinary tract in certain kidney diseases, with the use of certain diuretics, or with increased amounts of adrenal cortical steroid hormones (such as cortisone preparations).

Hypokalemia may occur through the increased urinary excretion of potassium caused by

kidney disease   **a** _____

certain diuretics   **b** _____

adrenal cortical hormones   **c** _____

373 The nurse will assess for signs and symptoms of low potassium in persons who are likely to develop a deficit. The clinical signs and symptoms of hypokalemia are not specific and may occur in seriously ill patients who do not have low serum potassium.[8] Potassium depletion may be evidenced by neuromuscular signs that include muscular cramps, paresthesias, muscular weakness progressing to flaccid paralysis, fatigue, and mental confusion.

The neuromuscular signs of hypokalemia include

cramps **a** paresthesias and muscle _____

flaccid paralysis **b** muscular weakness that may progress to _____
_____

confusion **c** fatigue and mental (alertness? confusion?)

374 The gastrointestinal signs of hypokalemia result from a reduction of neuromuscular irritability and a weakness of the smooth muscles of the gastrointestinal tract. Therefore a low level of potassium in the body may cause anorexia, abdominal distention, and paralytic ileus (absent peristalsis).

Hypokalemia may cause the following gastrointestinal signs:

anorexia **a** _____

abdominal distention **b** _____

paralytic ileus **c** _____

375 The most important abnormality of renal function when the level of potassium in the body is low is the inability of the kidneys to concentrate urine. Therefore the quantity of urine is increased.

When the level of potassium in the body is low, the
increased output of urine is (increased? unaffected? decreased?).

376 Extreme depletion of potassium involves the respiratory muscles. The diaphragm may be paralyzed. Respirations will become shallow, and death may result from apnea and respiratory arrest.

shallow A severe deficit in potassium will cause (shallow? deep?) respirations.

377 The cardiac signs of hypokalemia include irregular rhythm, heart block, altered electrocardiograph (ECG) patterns, circulatory failure, hypotension, and systolic arrest.

Hypokalemia may cause cardiac signs that include

irregular **a** (regular? irregular?) rhythm

abnormal **b** (normal? abnormal?) ECG patterns

arrest **c** circulatory failure, hypotension, and systolic _____

378 A deficit in potassium will affect repolarization, which is evident on the ECG. In general, the ECG changes include a shortened and depressed S-T segment, a flattened or inverted T wave, a prolonged Q-T interval, and a U wave that is equal to or higher than the T wave.

flat

a In hypokalemia the T wave is (flat? peaked?).

lengthened

b The Q-T interval is (shortened? lengthened?).

present

c A U wave is (present? absent?).

379 The normal serum potassium level varies from 3.5 to 5 mEq/L in adults. The range is slightly narrower in children (see p. 129). When the serum potassium level is 3 mEq/L or lower, signs of hypokalemia may become evident. We must remember that the serum potassium level does not tell us the total body potassium level.

3.5; 5

a Normal serum potassium levels in adults vary between _____ and _____ mEq/L.

3

b Signs of hypokalemia may occur when the serum potassium level is _____ mEq/L or lower.

380 If the hypokalemia is severe, laboratory tests will indicate metabolic alkalosis.

alkalosis

In severe hypokalemia the laboratory tests will indicate metabolic (acidosis? alkalosis?).

381 A deficit in potassium enhances the action of digitalis. Therefore if digitalis is given to a person with hypokalemia, digitalis toxicity is more likely to occur.

low

A toxic reaction to digitalis is more likely to occur if the potassium is (high? normal? low?).

382 Treatment of hypokalemia is aimed at replacing the potassium that has been lost. Potassium can be given intravenously to achieve a quick response. Potassium given orally is also effective. However, the most natural way to replace potassium is through a high-potassium diet. Many foods contain potassium. Fruit juices (especially orange juice), bananas, bouillon, and meat broths are rich sources.

Foods rich in potassium include

orange juice

a _____

bananas

b _____

bouillon

c _____

meat broths

d _____

383 If potassium is to be replaced by oral medication, there are several forms that may be used: potassium chloride, potassium citrate, potassium gluconate (Kaon), or combinations of these. Potassium-containing medications must be administered with caution because hyperkalemia can result from excessive dosages. Oliguria is an important sign of toxicity when potassium supplements are given.

decreased

A sign to be watched for when potassium medications are being administered is (increased? decreased?) urinary output.

384 There is no formula for calculating the amount of potassium needed to replace that which is lost, since most of the body's potassium is intracellular. Average deficits are in amounts of 200 to 400 mEq. However, the deficit may be as much as 800 to 1000 mEq of potassium.[8]

200; 1000

The range of deficit may be from _____ to _____ mEq of potassium.

385 If potassium is given intravenously, the rate must be limited. Forty milliequivalents of potassium should be diluted in 1000 ml of intravenous fluid for an adult. When potassium is given intravenously to an adult, the rate of infusion should not exceed 20 mEq/hr.[8] When potassium is given to a child through a peripheral vein, the concentration should not exceed 30 to 40 mEq/L. Potassium supplements for a child are usually calculated at approximately 2 to 4 mEq/kg/24 hr.[12]

a When potassium chloride is given intravenously to an

20

adult, it must be diluted and given at a rate of not more than _____ mEq of potassium per hour.

b When potassium is given intravenously to a child, the

weight

usual dose is calculated according to the _____ of the child.

386 The reason why potassium-containing solutions should not be given too rapidly intravenously is that the heart muscle is very sensitive to extracellular potassium. If the concentration of potassium rises too rapidly, cardiac arrest may occur. When potassium is administered intravenously, the patient must be observed for symptoms of hyperkalemia. (Hyperkalemia will be discussed later—frames 388 to 404.)

If intravenous potassium is administered too rapidly, death may occur from cardiac _____.

arrest

387 If the potassium is very low, the nurse could use the categories of either impaired physical mobility or of self-care deficit to begin a nursing diagnosis.

The nursing diagnostic category of impaired physical mobility or of self-care deficit could be appropriate in potassium deficit, since muscular weakness can progress to _____.

flaccid paralysis

SUMMARY

Potassium is the major cation in the intracellular fluid. It is necessary to maintain the volume of fluid within the cell, to regulate neuromuscular irritability, and to maintain the hydrogen ion concentration in the body. Normally potassium is ingested with the diet and excreted by the kidneys. Normal kidneys will continue to excrete potassium even with inadequate intake, however, so the regulation of potassium excretion depends on the amount of sodium available for exchange, the number of hydrogen ions being excreted, and the aldosterone level.

Clinically we do not measure the intracellular potassium; therefore the serum potassium level that is measured may not represent accurately the total body potassium. A low serum potassium is associated with alkalosis. Hypokalemia may be caused by a decreased intake or an increased output of potassium.

Depletion of potassium may occur when gastrointestinal secretions are lost through vomiting, gastric suction, intestinal fistulas, or diarrhea. Certain diseases of the kidney, treatment with diuretics, or increased adrenal cortical steroid hormones may also cause hypokalemia.

The clinical signs and symptoms of hypokalemia are

not specific but include neuromuscular signs of muscle cramps, paresthesias, muscular weakness progressing to paralysis, fatigue, and mental confusion. The gastrointestinal signs of hypokalemia include anorexia, abdominal distention, and paralytic ileus. The kidneys are unable to concentrate urine. The respirations become shallow, and death may result from apnea and respiratory arrest. The cardiac signs include irregular rhythm, heart block, altered ECG patterns, circulatory failure, hypotension, and systolic arrest. The normal serum potassium level is 3.5 to 5 mEq/L in an adult and 3.4 to 4.7 mEq/L in a child. The treatment of hypokalemia is replacement of the potassium.

REVIEW

potassium

1 The major intracellular cation is _____.

will

2 The kidneys (will? will not?) continue to excrete potassium when the intake of potassium is low.

3 Depletion of potassium may occur when gastrointestinal secretions are lost through any of the following:

vomiting   **a** _____

gastric suction   **b** _____

intestinal fistulas   **c** _____

diarrhea   **d** _____

are not

4 Clinical signs and symptoms of hypokalemia (are? are not?) specific.

paralysis

5 One of the symptoms of hypokalemia is muscular weakness that may progress to _____.

3.5 to 5

6 The normal serum potassium level for adults is _____ mEq/L.

is not

7 The serum potassium level (is? is not?) always an accurate picture of the total body potassium level.

8 Which of the following will have a greater loss of potassium?

142

√   _____ **a** A person taking a diuretic

_____ **b** A person taking a laxative

Potassium excess

388 Since normally functioning kidneys excrete potassium, abnormal potassium accumulation does not occur often. However, hyperpotassemia (or hyperkalemia), which is extremely dangerous, can occur from excessive parenteral administration or overly rapid administration of solutions containing potassium.

does not occur   **a** Hyperkalemia (occurs? does not occur?) frequently.

hyper-   **b** Excessive parenteral administration of potassium can cause (hyper-? hypo-?)kalemia.

389 Trauma to tissues (such as crush injuries) will liberate intracellular potassium and result in hyperkalemia.

crush   Intracellular potassium may be liberated by tissue trauma such as occurs in _____ injuries.

390 Adrenal cortical insufficiency will cause hyperkalemia. For example, in Addison's disease, in which aldosterone is lacking, potassium is not excreted normally. Therefore the level of potassium in the body goes up.

insufficiency   Adrenal cortical (insufficiency? overactivity?) will cause hyperkalemia.

391 Respiratory or metabolic acidosis may cause the serum potassium level to rise. In acidosis the hydrogen ion concentration in the extracellular fluid increases. This causes potassium to move out of the cells; then hydrogen and sodium ions move into the cell. Therefore the level of potassium in the serum increases.

hyper-   **a** Acidosis may cause (hypo-? hyper-?)kalemia.

hypo-   **b** Alkalosis may cause (hypo-? hyper-?)kalemia.

392 In a patient with renal failure, the serum level of potassium may be difficult to control. Hyperkalemia is more likely to occur after the urinary output falls below 400 to 500 ml/day in an adult.[8]

hyper-   In renal failure with a decreased urinary output, (hyper-? hypo-?)kalemia may occur.

143

393 Some of the more common causes of hyperkalemia include excessive administration of potassium, tissue trauma that liberates intracellular potassium, adrenal cortical insufficiency, acidosis, and renal failure with decreased urinary output. The major danger of hyperkalemia is its effect on the myocardium.

The danger of hyperkalemia is the effect on the
heart (myocardium) _____.

394 Hyperkalemia is a medical emergency because of its effect on the heart. The danger is that the patient will die of cardiac standstill. When the extracellular potassium is elevated to 7 mEq/L or more, heart block and ventricular standstill may occur.[18] When complete heart block is associated with hyperkalemia, the rate may be slow and the heart is in danger of stopping in diastole.

3.5 to 5   **a** Normal serum potassium in adults is _____ mEq/L.
b Heart block or ventricular standstill may occur when
7   the serum potassium is elevated to _____ mEq/L or more.

395 Neuromuscular symptoms of hyperkalemia include weakness that may progress to flaccid paralysis. Respiratory paralysis and involvement of the muscles of phonation may occur. Both hypokalemia and severe hyperkalemia may cause muscle paralysis. Movement of potassium and sodium is necessary for polarization and the spread of stimuli along the muscle fibers. If either persistent increased or decreased polarization occurs, the spread of the stimuli is blocked along the muscle fibers and muscle weakness or paralysis follows.

Muscle weakness or paralysis is a symptom of
both hypo- and hyper-   (hypo-? hyper-? both hypo- and hyper-?)kalemia.

396 Both hypokalemia and hyperkalemia may cause muscle weakness and paralysis. Paresthesias, or numbness and tingling sensations, are common in hyperkalemia. Paresthesias caused by hyperkalemia usually affect the face, tongue, hands, and feet.[8]

Paresthesias of the face, tongue, hands, and feet
hyper-   may be the result of (hypo-? hyper-?)kalemia.

144

397 The ECG changes in hyperkalemia include tall peaked T waves, widening of the QRS complex, and shortening of the Q-T interval. This is just the reverse of the ECG changes that occur in hypokalemia. Later the P-R interval becomes prolonged, and then the P waves flatten or disappear.

ECG changes that occur in hyperkalemia include the following:

tall peaked

shortened

P

a T waves are ＿＿＿＿＿＿＿ .

b Q-T interval is (shortened? lengthened?).

c The ＿＿＿＿ wave disappears.

398 The laboratory findings in hyperkalemia include a serum potassium of 6 mEq/L or higher.

3.5 to 5

6

a The normal serum potassium level is ＿＿＿＿ mEq/L in adults.

b Serum potassium levels of ＿＿＿＿ mEq/L or higher are present in hyperkalemia.

399 Other laboratory findings would be respiratory or metabolic acidosis. Hyperkalemia occurs in both respiratory and metabolic acidosis and is probably a compensatory mechanism. In acidosis the hydrogen ion concentration of the extracellular fluid increases. The potassium ions move out of the cells and into the extracellular fluid, and hydrogen and sodium ions move into the cells.[8]

acidosis

In hyperkalemia laboratory findings of respiratory or metabolic (acidosis? alkalosis?) may be present.

400 The aim of treatment is to find the cause and correct it when possible. The method used to treat hyperkalemia will depend on the cause and severity of the hyperkalemia and on the patient's homeostatic mechanisms. An uncomplicated excess of potassium can be treated by avoiding additional potassium intake either orally or parenterally. A serum potassium level of 6.5 mEq/L and an abnormal ECG are considered an emergency. The immediate treatment is aimed at inducing potassium to enter the cells. Hypertonic glucose may be given intravenously to help potassium shift from the extracellular fluid to the liver and muscle cells.

6.5

into

move into the cell

cells

gastrointestinal

peritoneal dialysis or
hemodialysis

a A serum potassium level of _____ mEq/L with an abnormal ECG is considered an emergency.

b Hypertonic glucose is given to help potassium move (into? out of?) cells.

401 Insulin is given with the glucose to induce the movement of potassium back into the cells. Sodium bicarbonate may be used to buffer the hydrogen ion and allow the potassium to return to the cells.

The use of glucose, insulin, and sodium bicarbonate is aimed at helping the potassium to _____ _____.

402 Calcium gluconate may be administered intravenously in the treatment of hyperkalemia to increase the movement of potassium ions into tissue cells. Testosterone may be administered to prevent excessive protein breakdown and facilitate diffusion of potassium into bone and tissue cells.

Both calcium gluconate and testosterone are useful in making possible the movement of potassium from the extracellular fluid into the _____ .

403 Drugs such as cation-exchange resins may be used to remove potassium from the body through the gastrointestinal tract. The cation-exchange resin, which is of the carboxylic acid type, gives up hydrogen ions for cations (e.g., potassium, sodium, calcium). The resin can be given orally or rectally. The resins may cause constipation or impaction, and a mild laxative may be necessary.

Cation-exchange resins may be used in the treatment of hyperkalemia and act to remove potassium by way of the _____ tract.

404 If these measures are not successful in lowering the serum potassium level, or if there is renal failure, the hyperkalemia should be treated by peritoneal dialysis or hemodialysis.

Hyperkalemia caused by renal failure should be treated by _____.

SUMMARY

Hyperkalemia does not occur often, since normal kidneys continue to excrete potassium even when the intake is not adequate. However, when it does occur, it may be caused by excessive parenteral administration of potassium, crush injuries, adrenal cortical insufficiency, and respiratory or metabolic acidosis. Another possible cause is renal failure with oliguria (decreased urinary output). The signs and symptoms of hyperkalemia are similar to those of hypokalemia except for the greater effect of hyperkalemia on the heart muscle.

Heart block and ventricular standstill may occur if the extracellular potassium is 7 mEq/L or more. Muscle weakness and paralysis are symptoms of both hypokalemia and hyperkalemia. Paresthesias caused by hyperkalemia usually affect the face, tongue, hands, and feet.

In hyperkalemia the ECG changes include tall peaked T waves, widening of the QRS complex, and a shortened Q-T interval. The P-R interval becomes prolonged, and then the P waves flatten or disappear. A serum potassium level of 6 mEq/L or more is present in hyperkalemia. The immediate treatment is aimed at inducing potassium to enter the cells.

REVIEW

Hyperkalemia

1 _____ may be caused by excessive administration of potassium.

insufficiency

2 Crush injuries and adrenal cortical (insufficiency? overactivity?) may cause hyperkalemia.

acidosis

3 Hyperkalemia may be caused by respiratory or metabolic (acidosis? alkalosis?).

low

4 In a person with renal failure, hyperkalemia is more likely to occur when the urinary output is (high? low?).

6

5 A serum potassium level of _____ mEq/L or more is present in hyperkalemia.

147

CASE STUDY

Cindy Jackson

1 Cindy Jackson has been admitted to the hospital complaining of increasing weakness. Ms. Jackson has multiple sclerosis, but she has been living alone and had been getting from her bed into her wheelchair by herself. Recently, she has been unable to even turn over in bed.

When her electrolyte report comes from the laboratory, you find the following: sodium, 139 mEq/L; potassium, 1 mEq/L; chloride, 96 mEq/L.

a Which of the electrolytes is the most abnormal?

potassium
_____

b With a very low potassium you would expect to find muscular _____.

weakness

c The most likely cause for Ms. Jackson's inability to turn over in bed is (exacerbation of her multiple sclerosis? low potassium?).

low potassium

2 You learn that her feet had been swelling and the physician had given her Lasix (diuretic) pills to take one per day. Recently the swelling has not gone down overnight, so she has been taking several extra Lasix tablets to reduce the swelling.

The explanation for Ms. Jackson's weakness is the low potassium caused by urinary (excretion? retention?) due to the Lasix without adequate intake of potassium.

excretion

3 With the data available, a possible nursing diagnosis could be knowledge deficit related to appropriate use of medication (Lasix) used for swelling of ankles as evidenced by muscle weakness and low serum potassium.

Ms. Jackson needs information about her _____ _____, _____, and _____.

medication;
signs; symptoms

MAGNESIUM IMBALANCE

405 Magnesium is the fourth most abundant cation in the body. Like potassium, most of the magnesium is intracellular. Therefore only small amounts of magnesium are present in the serum. Refer to the diagrams on page

13 to compare the amount of magnesium in the intracellular compartment with that in the intravascular and the interstitial compartments.

intracellular

a Most of the magnesium in the body is in the (intravascular? intracellular? interstitial?) compartment.

interstitial

b The smallest amount of magnesium is in the (intravascular? intracellular? interstitial?) compartment.

406 Approximately 50% of the total magnesium content of the body is present in bone. Only about 1% of the body's magnesium is in the extracellular fluid. The normal serum level of magnesium is 1.5 to 2.5 mEq/L in adults and 1.3 to 2.4 mEq/L in infants.

a The percent of magnesium that is extracellular is

1

_____.

1.5; 2.5

b The normal serum magnesium is _____ to _____ mEq/L in adults.

407 Magnesium has several essential functions. The importance of magnesium has been recognized more recently than that of some other electrolytes. Magnesium functions as an activator in many enzyme reactions. Some of the enzyme systems that magnesium activates are those that empower the B vitamins to function and those that are associated with carbohydrate and protein metabolism. Magnesium is required for the synthesis of nucleic acids and proteins.

enzyme

a Magnesium is necessary as an activator of many systems _____.

magnesium

b The synthesis of nucleic acid and proteins requires

_____.

408 Another function of magnesium is that it exerts an effect similar to that of calcium on neuromuscular function. At some points magnesium acts synergistically with calcium, while at others it is antagonistic. Magnesium affects skeletal muscle directly by depressing acetylcholine release at the synaptic junction. Therefore neuromuscular activity is increased when magnesium levels are decreased. Magnesium is commonly used to prevent convulsions in eclampsia (toxemia) of pregnancy.

When magnesium levels are increased, neuromuscular activity is (increased? decreased?).

decreased

409 So far we have seen that magnesium is essential as an activator in many enzyme reactions. It is especially necessary for carbohydrate metabolism, and it is required for the synthesis of nucleic acids and proteins. Magnesium affects neuromuscular functions; it also facilitates the transportation of sodium and potassium across cell membranes. If magnesium is deficient, the kidneys tend to excrete more potassium.

When magnesium is deficient, the kidneys are likely to excrete (more? less?) potassium.

more

410 Magnesium also influences the levels of intracellular calcium through its effect on parathyroid hormone secretions. If the level of magnesium in the body is below normal, the action of parathyroid hormone in maintaining normal serum calcium levels is impaired.

Magnesium influences the level of intracellular calcium by its effect on the secretion of _____ _____.

parathyroid hormone

411 Magnesium therefore functions as an activator in many enzyme reactions, in carbohydrate and protein metabolism, in the synthesis of nucleic acids and proteins, in neuromuscular function, and in the transportation of sodium and potassium across cell membranes, and it influences the levels of intracellular calcium. A healthy adult ingests about 25 mEq (180 to 300 mg) of magnesium per day, while a child requires 150 to 250 mg of magnesium per day. A major source of dietary magnesium is the chlorophyll in green vegetables.

a A major source of dietary magnesium is _____ _____.

chlorophyll in green vegetables

25

b A healthy adult ingests approximately _____ mEq of magnesium per day.

412 While a major source of magnesium is green vegetables, other foods also contain magnesium. It is abundant in nuts, legumes, and fruit such as bananas, grapefruit, and oranges. Magnesium is also plentiful in peanut butter and chocolate.

Which of the following foods contain abundant amounts of magnesium?

✓ _____ **a** Green beans

_____ **b** Milk

✓ _____ **c** Walnuts

_____ **d** Honey

✓ _____ **e** Peanut butter

413 Magnesium is absorbed from the intestine. A number of physiological factors influence normal absorption, including the total magnesium intake; the length of time it is in the intestine; the rate of water absorption; and the amounts of calcium, phosphate, and lactose in the diet. It is therefore understandable that persons who have had intestinal bypass surgery for obesity may develop magnesium deficiency.

diet

a Magnesium is usually taken into the body in the normal _____.

intestine

b Magnesium is absorbed from the _____.

414 Magnesium is lost from the body primarily in the urine. The kidneys are able to conserve magnesium ions, so that renal excretion may be less than 1 mEq/day on a magnesium-free diet, after a period of adjustment.

in the urine

a The major pathway for magnesium loss is _____

_____.

are

b The kidneys (are? are not?) able to conserve magnesium.

Magnesium deficit (hypomagnesemia)

415 We have considered the function, as well as the intake and loss, of magnesium. Most of the factors that control magnesium metabolism are not known.[8] The major site of regulation is probably intracellular, but its mechanism is unknown.[18] A low serum magnesium level is called hypomagnesemia. Hypomagnesemia is present when the serum concentration of magnesium is less than 1.5 mEq/L.

1.5; 2.5

a Normal serum magnesium is _____ to _____ mEq/L.

b Hypomagnesemia is present when the serum magnesium is less than _____ mEq/L.

1.5

416 Remember that only 1% of the magnesium in the body is extracellular. Therefore there is no direct correlation between serum concentration and the total body store of magnesium. Usually when symptoms are present, the serum magnesium concentration will be below 1 mEq/L.

When symptoms of hypomagnesemia are present, the serum magnesium usually will be below _____ mEq/L.

1

417 A deficit in magnesium is not usually a result of dietary restrictions. However, it can occur with prolonged malnutrition or starvation, or if a patient is given magnesium-free fluids intravenously along with no oral intake and/or with nasogastric suction. Persons receiving parenteral hyperalimentation (total parenteral nutrition) in which there is inadequate magnesium may develop hypomagnesemia.

a An inadequate intake of magnesium will lead to

hypomagnesemia

_____.

do

b Persons who are receiving no oral intake (do? do not?) need magnesium added to the intravenous fluids.

418 Hypomagnesemia can be caused by inadequate intake, as discussed in frame 417. A more common cause is impaired intestinal absorption.

Impaired intestinal absorption of magnesium will

hypomagnesemia

lead to _____.

419 Children or adults with malabsorption syndrome (nontropical sprue or steatorrhea) or chronic diarrhea may develop hypomagnesemia. Persons with gastrointestinal fistulas may also develop hypomagnesemia. In these persons magnesium is excreted in the stool in the form of magnesium soaps.

Persons with malabsorption syndrome or chronic diarrhea may develop (hyper-? hypo-?) magnesemia.

hypo-

420 Another cause of hypomagnesemia is an excessive

intake of calcium, which impairs magnesium absorption, since they compete for the same absorption site.

Hypomagnesemia may be caused by an excessive intake of _____.

calcium

421 Magnesium deficit can be induced by alcoholism. Alcohol ingestion seems to promote a magnesium deficit that is unrelated to dietary intake.[31]

Alcohol ingestion seems to promote a magnesium (deficit? excess?).

deficit

422 Other causes of impaired absorption of magnesium include bowel resection, small bowel bypass, or inherited intestinal defects in magnesium absorption.

Bowel resection may contribute to a magnesium (deficit? excess?).

deficit

423 We have considered inadequate intake of magnesium and impaired absorption as causes of hypomagnesemia. Other causes of hypomagnesemia include excessive renal excretion or fluid loss.

Three categories of causes of hypomagnesemia include

inadequate intake

a _____

impaired absorption

b _____

excessive loss

c _____

424 The usual cause of excessive renal excretion of magnesium is diuretic therapy. Hypomagnesemia may be clinically significant when produced by diuretic therapy because many of these persons are also taking digitalis. There is evidence that digitalis toxicity can be aggravated by hypomagnesemia.

A common cause of excessive renal excretion of magnesium is _____ therapy.

diuretic

425 Another cause of hypomagnesemia is major surgery. Following major surgery, excessive urinary loss of magnesium occurs for 24 hours.

During the first 24 hours following major surgery, excessive urinary (loss? retention?) of magnesium occurs.

loss

426 Increased magnesium loss also occurs in diabetic ketoacidosis, primary aldosteronism, primary hyperparathyroidism, and other hypercalcemic states.

increased

In diabetic ketoacidosis (increased? decreased?) magnesium loss occurs.

427 Excessive urinary excretion of magnesium may occur with several types of renal disease.

magnesium

Renal disease may cause increased urinary excretion of _____.

428 In considering excessive renal loss of magnesium we have included diuretic therapy, major surgery, diabetic ketoacidosis, primary aldosteronism, primary hyperparathyroidism, and other hypercalcemic states, as well as renal disease. Hypomagnesemia may also occur in hypoparathyroidism in association with hypocalcemia. Whenever hypocalcemia and hypokalemia exist, expect to find hypomagnesemia.

low

When a person has a low calcium and a low potassium level, you should expect to find a (high? low?) level of magnesium.

429 We have seen that hypomagnesemia may be caused by inadequate intake, impaired absorption, or excessive renal excretion. Although the clinical picture varies from patient to patient, the nurse will assess for certain signs and symptoms that are frequently seen. Remember that one of the actions of magnesium is its effect on neuromuscular function. The signs and symptoms of magnesium deficit are characterized by neuromuscular irritability; these include tremor, athetoid or choreiform movements (slow, involuntary twisting and writhing movements), tetany, increased reflexes, clonus, a positive Babinski's sign, a positive Chvostek's sign, paresthesias of the feet and legs, excessive neuromuscular irritability, and convulsions.

A positive Babinski's sign is the dorsiflexion of the great toe with fanning of the other toes when the lateral aspect of the sole is stroked sharply. However, in an infant this is a normal response up until about age 2 years. Chvostek's sign is elicited by tapping the person's face just in front of the ear over the facial nerve. Tapping over the nerve will cause unilateral spasm of the lip, nose, or eyelid when the test is positive.

a The signs and symptoms of magnesium deficit are characterized by neuromuscular _____ .

irritability

b Which of the following are signs or symptoms of magnesium deficit?

√ _____ (1) Tremor

_____ (2) Negative Babinski's sign

√ _____ (3) Tetany

√ _____ (4) Increased reflexes

_____ (5) Lethargy

√ _____ (6) Convulsions

430 Other signs and symptoms of magnesium deficit include personality changes with agitation, mental depression or confusion, and hallucinations, which are usually auditory or visual.

A person who develops a personality change with agitation or becomes mentally depressed or confused or

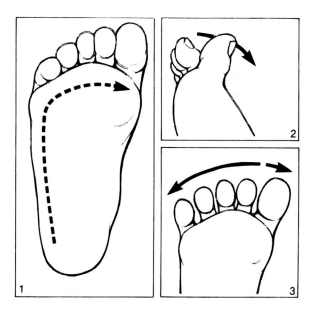

Babinski's reflex. 1, Direction of stroke. 2, Dorsiflexion of big toe. 3, Fanning of toes. (From Whaley LF and Wong DL: Nursing care of infants and children, *ed. 4, St. Louis, 1991, Mosby–Year Book.)*

deficit

develops hallucinations may have a magnesium (deficit? excess?).

431 There may be cardiovascular signs of a magnesium deficit, including tachycardia with atrial or ventricular premature contractions, and nonspecific T wave changes in the electrocardiogram.

Which of the following signs may result from magnesium deficit?

_____ **a** Bradycardia

√ _____ **b** Atrial or ventricular premature contractions

√ _____ **c** Nonspecific T wave changes

432 Most of the signs and symptoms of a magnesium deficit are related to the neuromuscular, neurological, or cardiovascular systems. Hypomagnesemia and hypocalcemia may coexist. This is especially true in persons with an excessive loss of gastrointestinal fluids.

neurological
neuromuscular
cardiovascular
hypo-

a Most of the signs and symptoms of a magnesium deficit are related to the _____, _____ , and _____ systems.

b When hypocalcemia is present, (hyper-? hypo-?) magnesemia may also be present.

433 Hypomagnesemia and hypercalcemia may also coexist in hyperparathyroid persons and in persons who have neoplastic disease with osteolytic metastasis (metastasis to bone).

hyper-

In persons with hyperparathyroid function or who have neoplastic disease with metastasis to bone, hypomagnesemia may coexist with (hypo-? hyper-?)calcemia.

434 A deficit in magnesium may precipitate or aggravate digitalis toxicity.

low

A toxic reaction to digitalis is more likely to occur if the serum magnesium is (high? low?).

435 Treatment of hypomagnesemia consists of correcting the underlying cause of the low serum magnesium intravenously, intramuscularly, or orally with magne-

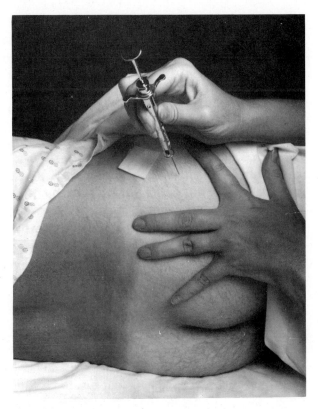

From Perry AG and Potter PA: Clinical nursing skills and techniques, *ed. 2, St. Louis, 1991, Mosby–Year Book.*

sium salts. Magnesium sulfate is the most commonly used magnesium salt.

correcting the cause

a Hypomagnesemia should be treated by first _____ _____.

magnesium sulfate

b The most commonly used magnesium salt is _____ _____.

436 Magnesium salts can be given orally to counteract continuous excessive losses. When magnesium is given orally, diarrhea is a possible side effect.

diarrhea

A possible side effect of magnesium salts given orally is _____.

437 In an adult magnesium sulfate can be given intramuscularly in a dose of 2 g (16.3 mEq) every 8 hours for 3 to 5 days. Repeated intramuscular injections should be given at different sites because the injections may be painful. Procaine hydrochloride 1% can be added to the injection if a large dose is used.

Intramuscular injections of magnesium sulfate are (likely? not likely?) to be painful.

likely

438 In an adult magnesium sulfate can also be given intravenously when hypomagnesemia is severe and may be associated with convulsions. In an adult, when magnesium is given intravenously, it must not exceed a rate of 150 mg/min. A rate of 1.5 ml/min of a 10% solution or 3 ml/min of a 5% solution should not be exceeded for an adult.

a The maximum safe rate for giving magnesium intravenously in an adult is _____ mg/min.

150

b If you are giving a 10% solution of magnesium, the maximum safe rate is _____ ml/min for an adult.

1.5

439 During an intravenous infusion of magnesium sulfate, the patient should not be left alone. You should observe the effectiveness of the magnesium infusion in relieving signs and symptoms. Observe for the anticonvulsant effect, relaxation of spastic muscles, and resolution of tremors and arrhythmias.

Signs indicating that the magnesium infusion is effective include a decrease in

muscle tension **a** _____

tremors **b** _____

arrhythmias **c** _____

440 Whenever magnesium sulfate is given intravenously, you must monitor the patient for signs and symptoms of high serum magnesium (see frames 453 to 457). Check every 5 minutes or before each dose for flaccidity and loss of patellar (knee-jerk) reflex.

a When giving magnesium sulfate intravenously, you must monitor the patient for signs of (high? low?) serum magnesium.

high

b You should check for loss of the patellar reflex every _____ minutes.

5

441 In addition to checking for loss of the patellar reflex, you should also count the respiratory rate every 5 minutes. Be sure the respiratory rate is at least 16/min. Respiratory paralysis may occur during infusion of magnesium sulfate.

During intravenous infusion of magnesium sulfate, you should check for _____ and _____ every 5 minutes.

loss of patellar reflex
respiratory rate

442 During intravenous infusion of magnesium sulfate, you should look for flushing of the skin, especially of the face, and for diaphoresis.

Observations to be made during an intravenous infusion of magnesium sulfate include (redness? paleness?) of the face and (moist? dry?) skin.

redness
moist

443 In addition to checking reflexes, respiratory rate, and condition of the skin, you need to check the blood pressure of the person receiving magnesium sulfate intravenously. During an infusion, you should check the patient's blood pressure every 5 to 10 minutes to detect hypotension.

During infusion of magnesium sulfate, the blood pressure should be checked every _____ to _____ minutes.

5; 10

444 When giving intravenous infusion of magnesium sulfate, you should slow or stop the infusion and notify the physician if any one of the following signs appears: loss of the patellar reflex, decreased respiratory rate,

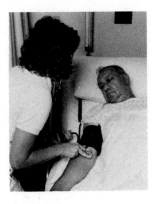

From Perry AG and Potter PA: Cliniucal nursing skills and techniques, ed. 2, St. Louis, 1991, Mosby–Year Book.

flushing of the face, diaphoresis, flaccidity, or hypotension.

During intravenous infusion of magnesium sulfate, you should slow or stop the infusion if which of the following signs appear?

√   _____ **a** Loss of the patellar reflex
              _____ **b** Increased respiratory rate of 24
√   _____ **c** Flushing of the face
              _____ **d** Spasticity
√   _____ **e** Hypotension

445 If magnesium levels become high, respiratory failure may occur (see frames 455 through 457).

If magnesium levels become high, you must be prepared to manage respiratory _____.

failure

446 One of the prime responsibilities of the nurse in caring for a person with a magnesium deficit is to provide for the patient's safety. Since convulsions may occur, protective measures must be taken to prevent injury.

Persons with a magnesium deficit must be protected from injury that could result during a _____.

convulsion

447 Another reason why persons with a magnesium deficit have special safety needs is that they may become confused and/or may develop hallucinations.

Persons with a magnesium deficit need to be protected, since they may become (drowsy? confused?) and may develop hallucinations.

confused

448 A category that could be used in writing a nursing diagnosis for a person with a magnesium deficit, who is being treated with intravenous magnesium would be potential for injury.

Potential for injury would be an appropriate category to use in writing a nursing diagnosis for a person with magnesium deficit who is being treated with _____ .

intravenous magnesium

SUMMARY

Magnesium is the second most abundant cation in the intracellular fluid. Magnesium is essential as an activator in many enzyme reactions, especially carbohydrate metabolism. It is required for the synthesis of nucleic acids and proteins, and it is important for normal neuromuscular function. It influences the levels of intracellular calcium and facilitates transportation of sodium and potassium across cell membranes.

Most of the magnesium is in the intracellular fluid. Only about 1% of magnesium is extracellular. Normal serum magnesium is 1.5 to 2.5 mEq/L.

Magnesium deficit may occur with prolonged malnutrition, starvation, alcoholism, or administration of magnesium-free intravenous fluids along with no oral intake. A deficit in magnesium may be caused by impaired intestinal absorption or loss through diarrhea or draining gastrointestinal fistulas. Excessive loss of magnesium may occur through renal excretion.

The clinical signs and symptoms of hypomagnesemia are not specific but may include mental changes such as personality change, agitation, mental depression, confusion, or hallucinations. The neuromuscular signs and symptoms include tremor, tetany, clonus, increased reflexes, positive Babinski's sign, positive Chvostek's sign, paresthesias, and convulsions. The cardiovascular signs and symptoms include tachycardia, atrial or ventricular premature contractions, and nonspecific T wave changes in the electrocardiogram.

REVIEW

magnesium

1 The second major intracellular cation is _____.

enzyme

2 Magnesium is essential as an activator in many _____ reactions.

1.5; 2.5

3 Normal serum magnesium is _____ to _____ mEq/L.

161

4 A magnesium deficit may result from inadequate intake such as

a _____

b _____

c _____

5 Excessive loss of magnesium may be caused by intestinal conditions such as

a _____

b _____

c _____

6 Clinical signs and symptoms of hypomagnesemia (are? are not?) specific.

are not

7 Personality change, confusion, or hallucinations may occur with (hypo-? hyper-?)magnesemia.

hypo-

8 Which of the following are neuromuscular signs and symptoms of hypomagnesemia?

√ _____ **a** Tremor

_____ **b** Depressed reflexes

√ _____ **c** Positive Babinski's sign

√ _____ **d** Convulsions

Magnesium excess

449 Magnesium excess, or hypermagnesemia, is not a common imbalance. Hypermagnesemia seldom develops except in renal failure.

The most common cause of hypermagnesemia

renal failure is _____.

450 Hypermagnesemia is a serum magnesium level over 2.5 mEq/L.

1.5; 2.5 **a** Normal serum magnesium in adults is _____ to _____ mEq/L.

b A serum magnesium level of 3 mEq/L would be

hypermagnesemia called _____ .

451 While renal failure is the most common cause of hypermagnesemia, excessive use of magnesium-containing medications can also contribute to hypermagnesemia. A person with renal failure who takes large amounts of magnesium-containing antacids or cathartics may develop hypermagnesemia.

hyper-

A person who takes large amounts of magnesium-containing antacids may develop (hyper-? hypo-?) magnesemia.

452 Hypermagnesemia occurs in a person with diabetic ketoacidosis when there has been severe water loss.

hypermagnesemia

A person who has diabetic ketoacidosis with severe dehydration may develop _____.

453 The signs and symptoms of hypermagnesemia will vary with the level of serum magnesium. When the serum magnesium is between 3 and 5 mEq/L, the vasodilating effect of magnesium can cause hypotension. Flushing, a feeling of warmth, and diaphoresis may also occur.

3; 5

A patient with a serum magnesium of _____ to _____ mEq/L may have hypotension.

454 When the serum magnesium increases to a level of 5 to 7 mEq/L, the person becomes drowsy. At a serum magnesium level of 7 mEq/L, the deep tendon reflexes are lost.[8]

5

a A person may become drowsy when the serum magnesium is over _____ mEq/L.

absent

b When the serum magnesium level is 7 mEq/L, the deep tendon reflexes are (increased? decreased? absent?).

455 The respiratory center is depressed when the serum magnesium rises to 10 mEq/L.[8]

10

Respiratory depression occurs at a serum level of _____ mEq/L.

456 Coma may occur at serum magnesium levels of 12 to 15 mEq/L, and cardiac arrest is likely at concentrations of 15 to 20 mEq/L.[8]

cardiac

At serum magnesium levels over 15 mEq/L, coma is likely to occur, followed by _____ arrest.

457 The sequence of the signs and symptoms of increasing magnesemia are hypotension, drowsiness, loss of deep tendon reflexes, respiratory depression, coma, and cardiac arrest.

Loss of deep tendon reflexes is likely to occur at a serum magnesium level of _____ mEq/L.

7

458 Intervention is aimed at treating the cause of the magnesium excess. Magnesium salts should not be given to persons with renal failure. If renal failure is present, dialysis will likely be necessary even though dialysis is not very efficient in removing magnesium.

should not

Persons with renal failure (should? should not?) take medications containing magnesium salts.

459 Another useful treatment for hypermagnesemia is the use of intravenous calcium gluconate. Calcium has an antagonistic effect on magnesium and can therefore be a useful temporary measure. (See frame 504 for calcium infusions.)

An electrolyte that has an antagonistic effect on magnesium and may be used in treating hypermag-

calcium

nesemia is _____.

460 The nurse must assess patients for signs and symptoms that would indicate possible increasing hypermagnesemia.

The first step in the nursing care of patients with po-

assessment

tential hypermagnesemia is _____ .

SUMMARY

Hypermagnesemia seldom occurs except in persons with renal failure. A serum level of magnesium over 2.5 mEq/L is hypermagnesemia. Excessive use of magnesium-containing medications by a person with renal failure can contribute to hypermagnesemia. Persons with diabetic ketoacidosis and severe water loss may develop hypermagnesemia. The progression of signs and symptoms of hypermagnesemia is from hypotension, flushing, diaphoresis, drowsiness, loss of deep tendon reflexes, and respiratory depression to coma and cardiac arrest.

REVIEW

hypermagnesemia

1 A serum magnesium of 3 mEq/L is _____.

renal failure

2 The most common cause of hypermagnesemia is _____ .

hypotension

3 One of the earliest signs of hypermagnesemia is _____ .

absent

4 At a serum magnesium level of 7 mEq/L, deep tendon reflexes are likely to be _____.

antagonistic

5 Calcium gluconate is sometimes used in treating hypermagnesemia because calcium is _____ to magnesium.

CALCIUM IMBALANCE

461 Serum calcium imbalance can be a real medical emergency; therefore it is important for you to know how the body normally balances calcium and how to anticipate and recognize a calcium imbalance. Calcium is the most abundant cation in the body. However, 99% of the calcium is in the bones.

cation

Calcium is the most abundant (cation? anion?) in the body.

462 The other 1% of the calcium in the body is in the blood plasma or serum. The calcium concentration in the extracellular compartment normally remains remarkably constant. Normally the total serum calcium is in the range of 4.5 to 5.3 mEq/L or 9 to 10.6 mg/100 ml in adults and children.

1

a The amount of calcium in the serum is _____ %.

remains constant

b Normally the serum calcium concentration (remains constant? fluctuates widely?).

4.5 to 5.3

c The normal serum calcium concentration is (1.5 to 2.5? 3.5 to 5.0? 4.5 to 5.3?) mEq/L.

463 The calcium in the intravascular compartment is mainly in two forms: one form is ionized calcium, which is physiologically active; the second form is the calcium that is bound to protein.

a The form of calcium that is physiologically active is

ionized _____ calcium.

protein **b** The bound calcium in the blood is bound to _____ .

464 Normally 50% to 75% of the serum calcium is ionized.

active **a** Ionized serum calcium is physiologically (inactive? active?).

b The amount of serum calcium that is ionized is

50; 75 _____ % to _____%.

465 While 50% to 75% of the serum calcium is ionized, the rest is bound to protein. Most of the bound calcium is combined with albumin. The calcium that is bound to plasma protein cannot pass through the capillary wall and therefore cannot leave the intravascular compartment.

a Most of the calcium that is bound to protein is bound

albumin to _____.

cannot **b** Calcium that is bound to plasma protein (can? cannot?) pass through the capillary wall.

466 Clinically the serum calcium level can be misleading unless it is correlated with the serum albumin level. As the total protein in the blood decreases, less serum calcium is bound.

a The serum calcium level should be correlated with

albumin the serum _____ level.

less **b** When the total protein in the blood decreases, (more? less?) calcium is bound.

467 Any change in serum protein will result in a change in the total serum calcium. The amount of that change is about 0.8 mg/100 ml of serum calcium for each 1 g/100 ml of serum protein.

a decrease   A decrease in serum protein will result in (a decrease? an increase?) in serum calcium.

468 One of the functions of calcium, along with phosphorus, is to provide strength and durability to bones and teeth. As we learned earlier, 99% of the calcium is in the bones. While the serum calcium is a small percentage of the total, it is essential for some vital physiological processes.

strength; durability   **a** Calcium provides _____ and _____ to bones and teeth.

essential   **b** The calcium in the serum is (essential? nonessential?) for some of the vital physiological processes.

469 Free, ionized calcium is needed to help maintain the permeability of cell membranes. Calcium is essential for the transmission of nerve impulses and neuromuscular excitability, and it is necessary for normal cardiac function.

permeability   **a** Calcium is necessary to help maintain the _____ of cell membranes.

transmission   **b** Calcium is necessary for the _____ of nerve impulses.

470 In addition to helping maintain the permeability of cell membranes and influencing neuromuscular function, calcium is needed for blood coagulation.

needed   Calcium is (needed? not needed?) for blood coagulation.

471 Calcium is also important in activating enzyme reactions and hormone secretion.

activating   Calcium functions by _____ enzyme reactions.

472 Within the range that is compatible with life, fluctuations in the concentration of calcium greatly affect the excitability of nerve tissue. Nerve cell membranes are less excitable when sufficient calcium is available.

sedative   Calcium acts as a (sedative? stimulant?) on nerve cell membranes.

473 We have considered some of the functions of calcium. We will now look at the absorption of calcium. Our bodies have an exquisite control system for maintaining the level of calcium in the serum. The serum calcium comes from the resorption of bone, intestinal absorption, and renal tubular resorption.

List three sources of serum calcium:

bone resorption   **a** _____

intestinal absorption   **b** _____

renal resorption   **c** _____

474 Serum calcium is lost by bone deposition and by renal and gastrointestinal excretion.

deposition   **a** Serum calcium is decreased by bone (deposition? resorption?).

excretion   **b** Serum calcium is decreased by gastrointestinal (excretion? resorption?).

excretion   **c** Serum calcium is decreased by renal tubular (resorption? excretion?).

475 The serum calcium level is influenced by both the resorption and the formation of bone. Bone deposition or formation occurs in response to stress and strain.

deposition   Stress and strain on the skeleton results in bone (deposition? resorption?).

476 The major factors that control the serum calcium concentration are vitamin D, parathyroid hormone, calcitonin (thyrocalcitonin), and the serum concentrations of calcium and phosphate ions. Calcitonin (thyrocalcitonin) is a hormone that has a weak effect on extracellular calcium. Calcitonin is secreted by the thyroid gland and reduces the blood calcium concentration.

D   **a** The vitamin that is important in controlling the serum calcium concentration is _____.

parathyroid
calcitonin   **b** The two hormones that are important in the control of serum calcium concentration are _____ and _____.

weak   **c** Calcitonin has a (weak? strong?) effect on the serum calcium concentration.

phosphate   **d** The serum concentrations of calcium and _____ ions influence the serum calcium level.

477 Vitamin D, essential for regulating calcium, is ingested in food and is synthesized in the body.

Two sources of vitamin D are

food
a _____

synthesis in the body
b _____

478 The general actions of vitamin D are to increase calcium absorption from the gastrointestinal tract and to mobilize calcium ions from the bones.

a Absorption of calcium from the gastrointestinal tract is (increased? decreased?) by vitamin D.

increased

b Vitamin D mobilizes _____ ions from the bones.

calcium

479 In addition to vitamin D, parathyroid hormone is important in controlling the serum concentration of calcium. Parathyroid secretion is stimulated by a low serum calcium concentration.

Because of the feedback mechanism, a high serum calcium concentration would (stimulate? suppress?) parathyroid secretion.

suppress

480 One of the functions of parathyroid hormone is to stimulate calcium and phosphate resorption from bone. This would increase the serum calcium concentration.

Parathyroid hormone (stimulates? suppresses?) resorption of calcium and phosphate from bone.

stimulates

481 Parathyroid hormone stimulates resorption of bone, which involves breaking down bone to release calcium and phosphate. Parathyroid hormone also influences the serum calcium concentration through its effect on the kidney to increase the excretion of phosphate ions.

Parathyroid hormone (increases? decreases?) the renal excretion of phosphate ions.

increases

482 Parathyroid hormone reduces the amount of phosphate ions that are resorbed by the kidney tubules. Therefore more phosphate is excreted in the urine and the serum phosphate concentration falls.

a Parathyroid hormone influences the kidney tubules to resorb (more? less?) phosphate ions.

less

b When more phosphate is excreted, the serum phosphate concentration (falls? rises?).

falls

169

483 Generally speaking, as phosphate levels decrease, serum calcium levels increase.

Serum calcium levels increase as phosphate levels

decrease _____ .

484 So far we have considered the effect of vitamin D and of parathyroid hormone on serum calcium levels. Calcitonin inhibits calcium mobilization from bone and therefore tends to lower serum calcium levels in a way that is opposite that of parathyroid hormone. Calcitonin secretion is stimulated directly by a high serum calcium level.

decrease **a** The effect of calcitonin is to (increase? decrease?) serum calcium levels.

increase **b** The effect of parathyroid hormone is to (increase? decrease?) serum calcium levels.

opposite **c** Therefore the effect of calcitonin and of parathyroid hormone on the serum calcium level is (the same? opposite?).

Calcium deficit

485 A serum calcium deficit is called hypocalcemia. In hypocalcemia the serum calcium is below 4.5 mEq/L.

5.3 **a** Normal serum calcium is 4.5 to _____ mEq/L.

4.5 **b** In hypocalcemia, the serum calcium is below _____ mEq/L.

486 A serum calcium deficit can occur from inadequate intake or from decreased absorption from the intestine. Persons with pancreatic disease or disease of the small intestine may fail to absorb calcium and will then excrete large amounts of calcium in the feces.

a Serum calcium deficit can occur from inadequate

intake _____ .

hypo- **b** Decreased absorption of calcium from the intestine may result in (hypo-? hyper-?)calcemia.

487 Parathyroid hormone deficiency (hypoparathyroidism) or vitamin D deficiency may result in hypocalcemia. Parathyroid hormone deficiency may develop after thyroid or parathyroid surgery.

a deficit **a** Hypocalcemia may be caused by (an excess? a deficit?) of parathyroid hormone.

hypo-

b Vitamin D deficiency may result in (hypo-? hyper-?) calcemia.

488 Rapid dilution of the plasma by intravenous calcium-free solutions may result in hypocalcemia.

hypocalcemia

Giving intravenous fluids rapidly without calcium may result in _____.

489 We have looked at inadequate intake, decreased absorption, pancreatic disease, disease of the small intestine, parathyroid hormone deficiency, vitamin D deficiency, and rapid dilution of the plasma as possible causes of hypocalcemia.

Of the following, which may cause hypocalcemia?

√   _____ **a** Decreased intestinal absorption

√   _____ **b** Pancreatic disease

   _____ **c** Hyperactive parathyroids

√   _____ **d** Vitamin D deficiency

√   _____ **e** Calcium-free intravenous fluids

490 Other possible causes of hypocalcemia include magnesium deficiency and neoplastic diseases.

deficiency

a Hypocalcemia may be caused by magnesium (deficiency? excess?).

hypo-

b Neoplastic diseases may cause (hypo-? hyper-?)calcemia.

491 Another cause of hypocalcemia is renal insufficiency. When the kidneys are unable to excrete phosphorus normally, hyperphosphatemia results. When the phosphorus rises, the serum calcium level falls.

hypo-

When hyperphosphatemia occurs, (hyper-? hypo-?) calcemia follows.

492 The signs and symptoms of hypocalcemia include those associated with neural excitability. Tetany is the most characteristic sign of hypocalcemia.

tetany

A characteristic sign of hypocalcemia is _____.

493 The signs and symptoms of increased excitability include paresthesias, especially numbness or tingling; skeletal muscle cramps; abdominal spasms and cramps; hyperactive reflexes; and convulsions.

171

cramps

hyper-

a Neural excitability that occurs in hypocalcemia may be evidenced by skeletal and abdominal _____.

b Reflexes will be (hyper-? hypo-?)active.

494 Trousseau's sign may be present in persons with hypocalcemia. To test for Trousseau's sign, a blood pressure cuff is applied to the upper arm and the cuff is inflated above the systolic level for 3 minutes. A positive sign is the development of carpal spasm (see the illustration below). The person's thumb adducts, and the fingers contract.

hypo-

a Trousseau's sign may be present in persons with (hypo-? hyper-?)calcemia.

carpal spasm

b A positive Trousseau's sign is demonstrated by _____.

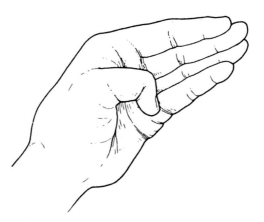

Carpal spasm. (From Groer MW: Physiology and pathophysiology of the body fluids, *St. Louis, 1981, The CV Mosby Co.)*

495 Chvostek's sign may also be used to observe an increase in neuromuscular excitability. Chvostek's sign is explained in frame 429.

an increase

A positive Chvostek's sign indicates (an increase? a decrease?) in neuromuscular excitability.

496 Mental changes occurring in hypocalcemia may include changes in mood, emotional depression, impairment of memory, confusion, or hallucinations.

Emotional depression or confusion may be evidenced in (hypo-? hyper-?)calcemia.

497 If the calcium deficit is prolonged, then calcium will be withdrawn from the bones to increase the extracellular calcium.

In a prolonged calcium deficit, calcium will be mobilized from _____.

498 It is well established that calcium absorption decreases with aging. The average elderly person in the United States is in negative calcium balance and is losing bone mass. There is growing evidence to indicate that the calcium intake may be inadequate.

a Calcium absorption (increases? decreases?) with aging.

b The average elderly person in the United States is in (negative? positive?) calcium balance.

499 By age 70, osteoporosis (loss of density of bone) may result in a decrease in skeletal height. The potential for pathological fractures is increased with osteoporosis. The structural change in skeletal mass may be related to a sedentary life-style, lack of exercise, low calcium intake, vitamin D deficiency, and excessive fat intake.

a When osteoporosis is present, the potential for pathological fractures is (increased? decreased?).

b The loss of skeletal mass (may? may not?) be related to the individual's life-style.

500 The current RDA (recommended dietary allowance) for calcium is 800 mg/day for children and adults and 1200 mg/day for adolescents. There is some evidence to suggest that this should be increased to 1200 to 1500 mg/day for the elderly.

a The current RDA for calcium for children and adults is _____ mg/day.

b The current RDA for calcium for adolescents is _____ mg/day.

c There is some evidence to suggest that the elderly should have a calcium intake of _____ to _____ mg/day.

501 In hypocalcemia a specific abnormal electrocardiographic finding is a prolonged Q-T interval.

An electrocardiographic finding that is characteristic of hypocalcemia is a prolonged _____ interval.

Q-T

502 It is important to observe for hypocalcemia in patients who have had recent surgery involving the thyroid or parathyroid glands. The serum calcium may drop rapidly and result in convulsions.

Following surgery involving the thyroid or parathyroid glands, patients should be observed for signs and symptoms of (hypo-? hyper-?)calcemia.

hypo-

503 Patients who are receiving total parenteral nutrition (hyperalimentation) or who are undergoing hemodialysis should be observed for signs and symptoms of hypocalcemia.

Hypocalcemia may develop in patients who are receiving _____ or who are undergoing _____ .

total parenteral nutrition
hemodialysis

504 Acute hypocalcemia is usually treated with a calcium salt, such as calcium gluconate, given intravenously. In cardiac arrest, 10 ml of a 10% solution (4.8 mEq) may be given within a 15- to 30-second period. In situations other than cardiac arrest, 10 ml of a 10% solution should not exceed 0.5 to 1.0 ml/min.

a The calcium salt preferred for treating acute hypocalcemia is _____.

calcium gluconate

b The intravenous rate for 10 ml of a 10% solution of calcium gluconate should not exceed _____ ml/min.

1

505 If the hypocalcemia is mild, a high-calcium diet or oral calcium salts may be given.

Calcium salts (may? may not?) be given orally in mild hypocalcemia.

may

506 In patients who are digitalized, calcium salts should be given cautiously and the patient must be observed continuously on a cardiac monitor. Calcium has an effect on the heart similar to that of digitalis. The arrhythmias that may occur include premature atrial or ventricular contractions, sinus bradycardia, and ventricular tachycardia.

a Calcium has an effect on the heart similar to that of

digitalis

_____.

b A digitalized patient must be observed on a cardiac

calcium

monitor when _____ salts are given intravenously.

507 Whenever calcium salts are being given, you must observe for the signs and symptoms of hypercalcemia. (See frames 517 through 526.)

hypercalcemia

Observe for signs and symptoms of _____ when calcium salts are being given.

SUMMARY

While calcium is the most abundant cation in the body, 99% of the calcium is in the bones. The 1% of calcium in the blood remains remarkably constant. The ionized calcium is needed to help maintain the permeability of cell membranes for the transmission of nerve impulses and neuromuscular excitability and for normal cardiac function. Also, calcium is necessary for blood coagulation, activating enzyme reactions, and hormone secretion.

Normally calcium is ingested with the diet and absorbed through the gastrointestinal tract. Serum calcium is gained by resorption of bone and by renal tubular resorption. Serum calcium is lost by renal and gastrointestinal excretion and by bone deposition. Major factors that control the serum calcium concentration are vitamin D, parathyroid hormone, calcitonin, and serum concentrations of calcium and phosphate ions.

A serum calcium deficit can occur from inadequate intake or from decreased absorption. Hypocalcemia may result from a deficiency of parathyroid hormone or of vitamin D. The signs and symptoms of hypocalcemia include those associated with neural excitability. Tetany is the most characteristic sign of hypocalcemia; therefore nursing care must include careful observation to detect increasing neuromuscular excitability. Hypocal-

175

cemia is usually treated with a calcium salt such as calcium gluconate.

REVIEW

calcium

1 The most abundant cation in the body is _____.

essential

2 Calcium is (essential? not essential?) for the transmission of nerve impulses.

tetany

3 The most characteristic sign of hypocalcemia is
_____ .

observation

4 In caring for a patient with a potential for hypocalcemia, an important nursing action is _____.

Calcium excess (hypercalcemia)

508 Hypercalcemia exists whenever the serum calcium
is over 5.3 mEq/L or 10.6 mg/100 ml.
a Hypocalcemia is indicated by a serum calcium level

4.5

below _____ mEq/L.

5.3

b A serum calcium level over _____ mEq/L indicates
hypercalcemia.

509 Hypercalcemia can be the result of excessive intake of calcium, excessive vitamin D intake, or conditions that promote the release of calcium from the
bones into the extracellular fluid.

excessive

a Hypercalcemia can result from (excessive? inadequate?) intake of calcium.

hyper-

b Excessive vitamin D intake can result in (hypo-? hy-
per-?)calcemia.

hypercalcemia

c Conditions that promote the release of calcium from
bones can result in _____.

510 Excessive calcium intake may occur with peptic
ulcer disease treated with milk and alkaline antacids,
especially calcium carbonate, for long periods.
A person with peptic ulcer disease who is treated
with milk and calcium carbonate may develop (hyper-?

hyper-

hypo-?)calcemia.

511 Hypercalcemia that develops from vitamin D over-dosage occurs primarily because of the increased absorption of calcium from the gastrointestinal tract.

Excessive vitamin D may result in hypercalcemia because of (increased? decreased?) absorption of calcium from the intestine.

increased

512 Several conditions may cause increased release of calcium from bones and thus result in hypercalcemia. The most common cause of hypercalcemia is cancer. Hypercalcemia can be a complication of almost any malignant disorder, but it is especially frequent in cancer of the breast. Bone metastasis may result in breakdown of normal bone and release of excessive calcium.

a Increased release of calcium from bone may cause (hypo? hyper-?)calcemia.

hyper-

b The most common cause of hypercalcemia is

cancer

_____ .

c Hypercalcemia is especially frequent in cancer of the

breast

_____.

513 While metastasis to bone may cause breakdown of bone and release of excessive calcium, cancer may cause hypercalcemia without bone metastasis. Many malignant tumors produce inappropriate hormones. Certain tumors produce a parathyroid-like substance, which causes increased bone resorption and a rise in the serum calcium concentration.

Causes of release of excessive calcium from bone:

metastasis

a cancer with _____ to bone

parathyroid

b production of a _____ -like hormone from the tumor

514 Bone destruction may exceed bone production to the extent that the kidneys are unable to excrete the excessive calcium ions. Also, hypercalcemia may result from a primary hyperparathyroidism, which may be caused by a benign adenoma of one or more parathyroid glands.

a Primary hyperparathyroidism may be caused by a

benign

_____ adenoma.

hyper-

b Hyperparathyroidism will result in (hypo-? hyper-?) calcemia.

515 Another cause of hypercalcemia is prolonged immobilization. Remember, we learned that bone deposition or formation occurs in response to stress and strain (frame 475). Therefore with disuse there is increased bone resorption, but bone formation is also decreased.

hyper-

a Prolonged immobilization may result in (hyper-? hypo-?)calcemia.

increased

b Disuse causes (increased? decreased?) bone resorption.

decreased

c Disuse results in (increased? decreased?) bone formation.

516 In considering the causes of hypercalcemia, we have looked at factors related to excessive intake of calcium, increased bone destruction, and decreased bone formation. There are other causes of hypercalcemia such as the use of diuretics, endocrine disorders, and renal diseases.

Factors that lead to hypercalcemia include the following:

√   _____ **a** Excessive intake of calcium

     _____ **b** Decreased bone destruction

√   _____ **c** Decreased bone formation

√   _____ **d** Use of diuretics

√   _____ **e** Renal diseases

517 The signs and symptoms of hypercalcemia result from three sources: a decrease in neuromuscular activity, resorption of calcium from bone, and the effect on the kidney of high calcium concentrations.

Three sources for the signs and symptoms of hypercalcemia include

a decrease

a (a decrease? an increase?) in neuromuscular activity

resorption

b (resorption? deposition?) of calcium from/in bone

high

c effect on the kidney of (high? low?) calcium concentration

518 The decreased neuromuscular activity will be evidenced in generalized muscle weakness, lethargy, loss of muscle tone, and ataxia. The person may show mental confusion, impairment of memory, slurred speech, personality or behavior changes, stupor, or coma.

a In hypercalcemia generalized muscle weakness results from the (increased? decreased?) neuromuscular activity.

decreased

b Stupor or coma may result from (hypo-? hyper-?)calcemia.

hyper-

519 The heart responds to hypercalcemia with effects that look like digitalis effect. Bradycardia and increased contractility occur in hypercalcemia. In the electrocardiogram, the Q-T interval shortens and the T waves invert. Ventricular arrhythmias may develop.

a Cardiac effects of hypercalcemia may include (brady-? tachy-?)cardia.

brady-

b The Q-T interval on the electrocardiogram (lengthens? shortens?).

shortens

c With hypercalcemia, ventricular _____ may develop.

arrhythmias

520 The gastrointestinal symptoms of hypercalcemia include anorexia, nausea, vomiting, and constipation.

Hypercalcemia may have symptoms including anorexia, nausea, vomiting, and (constipation? diarrhea?).

constipation

521 The signs and symptoms related to resorption of calcium from bone include deep bone pain and radiographic evidence of bone demineralization.

Deep bone pain may be caused by resorption of _____ from the bone.

calcium

522 High extracellular concentrations of calcium impair the ability of the kidney to concentrate urine.

When the kidney is less able to concentrate urine, (polyuria? anuria?) will be evident.

polyuria

523 The polyuria that results from hypercalcemia will lead to the need for increased intake of water.

Polyuria (will? will not?) lead to the need for increased water intake.

will

524 Hypercalcemia will predispose to the development of renal calculi (kidney stones).

Renal calculi may be the result of (hyper-? hypo-?) calcemia.

hyper-

525 Hypercalcemic crisis is an emergency condition caused by an acute increase in serum calcium levels above 8 to 9 mEq/L (17 mg/100 ml). Hypercalcemic crisis has signs and symptoms of intractable nausea, dehydration, stupor, and coma. Azotemia is present. Hypokalemia and/or hypomagnesemia may be present along with hypernatremia because of the water loss.

a Hypercalcemic crisis may occur if the serum calcium rises above _____ to _____ mEq/L.

8; 9

b The intractable nausea and vomiting will lead to a (deficit? excess?) in fluid volume.

deficit

c Another electrolyte imbalance likely to be present is (hypo-? hyper-?)kalemia.

hypo-

526 With hypercalcemic crisis, mortality has been high. Death often results from cardiac arrest.

high

Mortality is (high? low?) in hypercalcemic crisis.

527 Treating hypercalcemia involves removing the cause or controlling the condition that caused the excess serum calcium. When hypercalcemia is severe, the first thing to receive attention is the need for hydration. This will reduce the risk of renal damage and may reduce the serum calcium by dilution.

hydration

When hypercalcemia is severe, _____ must be adequate to reduce the possible renal damage.

528 Normal saline given intravenously will provide hydration, as well as produce some urinary excretion of calcium, since the kidneys selectively resorb sodium.

normal saline

The intravenous solution used to provide hydration in hypercalcemia is _____ .

529 When normal saline is given intravenously, it is important to match the rate and amount of saline solution to the patient's urine output. You need to measure the patient's hourly, as well as total, urine output.

hourly

When normal saline is given intravenously to treat hypercalcemia, you should measure the urine output _____ (frequency).

530 If normal saline does not produce adequate diuresis, then diuretics such as furosemide (Lasix) may be given to increase the excretion of calcium.

furosemide (Lasix)

Diuretics such as _____ may be used to increase the excretion of calcium.

531 Phosphate is used to lower the serum calcium level. Phosphate promotes deposition of calcium in bone and decreases intestinal absorption. A side effect of oral phosphate ingestion is diarrhea. Intravenous infusions of phosphate are used only for hypercalcemic crisis because of potential for soft tissue calcification and renal failure if the serum calcium decreases acutely.

phosphate

a The substance that acts by promoting deposition of calcium in bone and decreases intestinal absorption is _____.

hypercalcemic

b Intravenous infusions of phosphate are used only for _____ crisis.

532 Corticosteroids (Cortef) and mithramycin (Mithracin) are used for treating hypercalcemia in persons with cancer. Mithramycin is a potent antitumor drug that shares the cytotoxicities of other antitumor drugs but does lower serum calcium concentration.

cancer

Corticosteroids and mithramycin are used for treating hypercalcemia in persons with _____ .

533 In giving care to a person with hypercalcemia, it is important to protect him from pathological fractures. Positioning and moving must be done with extreme care to prevent fractures.

fractures

A potential problem for persons with hypercalcemia is pathological _____.

534 Formation of calcium stones in the urinary tract is another potential problem for persons with hypercalcemia. Persons with hypercalcemia should be encouraged to drink 3000 to 4000 ml of water per day to reduce the possibility of renal calculi.

calculi

a Persons with hypercalcemia may develop _____ in the urinary tract.

3000
4000

b Persons with hypercalcemia should drink _____ to _____ ml of water per day.

535 Acidic urine will help to decrease the possibility of urinary stone formation. Foods such as prunes or cranberry juice or ascorbic acid will favor increased acidity in the urine.

alkaline

a Urinary stone formation is more likely in (acidic? alkaline?) urine.

b Persons with hypercalcemia should eat foods that will help produce (acidic? alkaline?) urine.

acidic

536 Urinary tract infections should be avoided. Good perineal care and meticulous catheter care are especially important for persons with hypercalcemia.

infections

Good perineal care and meticulous catheter care will help prevent urinary tract _____ .

SUMMARY

Hypercalcemia can be the result of excessive calcium intake, excessive vitamin D intake, or conditions that promote release of calcium from the bones. Whenever bone destruction exceeds bone production to the extent that the kidneys are unable to excrete the excess calcium ions, hypercalcemia may result.

The signs and symptoms of hypercalcemia result from a decrease in neuromuscular activity, resorption of calcium from bone, and the effect on the kidney of high serum calcium concentrations. The decreased neuromuscular activity may be evidenced by generalized muscle weakness, loss of muscle tone, mental confusion, and coma. The cardiac signs of hypercalcemia include bradycardia, increased contractility, and ventricular arrhythmias. The increased resorption of bone is evidenced by deep bone pain and radiographic evidence of bone demineralization. The effect on the kidney is indicated by decreased concentration of urine, increased urine output, and renal calculi.

Hypercalcemic crisis is caused by a rapid increase in serum calcium levels to above 8 to 9 mEq/L. Adequate hydration must be provided. Diuretics and/or phosphate may be used to treat hypercalcemic crisis.

In caring for patients with hypercalcemia, it is important to protect them from pathological fractures. Urinary tract infections should be prevented. Intake of water should be in amounts of 3000 to 4000 ml/day.

REVIEW

1 Three causes of hypercalcemia include

excessive intake   **a** _____

excessive vitamin D   **b** _____

release of calcium from bone   **c** _____

a decrease   **2** The signs and symptoms of hypercalcemia include (a decrease? an increase?) in neuromuscular activity.

3 The increased resorption of bone is evidenced by

deep bone pain   **a** _____

radiographic evidence of demineralization   **b** _____

pathological fractures   **4** Patients with hypercalcemia should be moved gently because of the potential for _____.

3000; 4000   **5** A patient with hypercalcemia should have a daily fluid intake of _____ to _____ ml.

Normal values of electrolytes

Sodium	135-148 mEq/L
Potassium	3.5-5.0 mEq/L
Magnesium	1.5-2.5 mEq/L
Calcium	4.5-5.3 mEq/L

Assessment summary: fluids and electrolytes

Temperature
   Increased: sodium excess
   Decreased: sodium deficit, fluid volume deficit

Pulse
   Bounding, easily obliterated: fluid deficit
   Rapid, weak, thready: sodium deficit, fluid deficit
   Weak, irregular, rapid: potassium deficit
   Rapid: sodium excess

Respiration
   Deep, rapid: metabolic acidosis
   Shallow, slow, irregular: metabolic alkalosis
   Moist crackles: fluid excess
   Shallow breathing: potassium deficit
   Stridor: calcium deficit
   Depressed: magnesium deficit

Blood Pressure
   Hypotension: sodium deficit, potassium deficit, fluid deficit, magnesium deficit
   Hypertension: fluid excess, magnesium deficit
   Normal when lying flat and hypotension when head is elevated: fluid deficit

Skin and mucous membranes
   Poor skin turgor: fluid deficit
   Flushed, dry skin: sodium excess
   Cold, clammy skin: sodium deficit
   Finger printing on sternum: sodium deficit
   Rough, dry, red tongue: sodium excess
   Dry mucous membranes with longitudinal wrinkles on tongue: fluid deficit

Speech
   Difficulty forming words without first moistening tongue and lips: sodium excess, fluid deficit
   Hoarseness: fluid deficit
   Difficulty speaking because of muscular weakness: potassium deficit

Behavior
   Lassitude: fluid deficit, magnesium excess
   Impaired mental function: potassium deficit
   Apprehension and giddiness: sodium deficit
   Irritability, restlessness: potassium excess
   Excitement (maniacal): sodium excess
   Hallucinations: magnesium deficit

Assessment summary: fluids and electrolytes—cont'd

Skeletal muscles
   Hypotonus: potassium deficit, calcium excess
   Flabbiness: potassium deficit
   Flaccid paralysis: potassium deficit or excess
   Cramping of exercised muscles: calcium deficit
   Muscle rigidity: calcium deficit
   Chvostek's sign: calcium deficit, magnesium deficit
   Convulsions: magnesium deficit

Sensation
   Tingling of fingers and toes: calcium deficit, potassium
      deficit
   Light headed: respiratory alkalosis
   Abdominal cramps: sodium deficit, calcium deficit, potas-
      sium deficit
   Numb feeling: potassium deficit
   Deep bony flank pain: calcium excess
   Nausea: potassium excess, sodium deficit, calcium ex-
      cess
   Abnormal sensitivity to sound: magnesium deficit

Bibliography

1. Anthony CP and Thibodeau GA: Textbook of anatomy and physiology, ed 12, St. Louis, 1987, The CV Mosby Co.
2. Behrman RE and Vaughn VC: Nelson textbook of pediatrics, ed 13, Philadelphia, 1987, WB Saunders Co.
3. Beland IL: Clinical nursing, ed 4, New York, 1981, MacMillan Publishing Co.
4. Brocklehurst JC: Textbook of geriatric medicine and gerontology, ed 3, New York, 1985, Churchill Livingstone.
5. Brunner LS Emerson PE Jr, Ferguson LK, and Suddarth DS: Textbook of medical-surgical nursing, ed 6, Philadelphia, 1988, JB Lippincott Co.
6. Burke SR: The composition and function of body fluids, ed 3, St. Louis, 1980, The C.V. Mosby Co.
7. Ganong WF: Review of medical physiology, ed 13, Los Altos, Calif, 1987, Lange Medical Publications.
8. Goldberger EA: A primer of water, electrolyte and acid-base syndromes, ed 7, Philadelphia, 1986, Lea & Febiger.
9. Goodhart RS and Shils ME: Modern nutrition in health and disease, ed 6, Philadelphia, 1980, Lea & Febiger.
10. Groer MW: Physiology and pathophysiology of the body fluids, St. Louis, 1981, The CV Mosby Co.
11. Guyton AC: Textbook of medical physiology, ed 7, Philadelphia, 1986, WB Saunders Co.
12. Hazinski MF: Nursing care of the critically ill child, St. Louis, 1984, The CV Mosby Co.
13. Kaplan LC and Pesce AJ: Clinical chemistry: theory, analysis, and correlation, St. Louis, 1984, The CV Mosby Co.
14. Lentner C, editor: Geigy scientific tables, vol 1, units of measurement; body fluids; composition of the body; nutrition, ed 8, Summit, N.J., 1981, Ciba-Geigy Corp.
15. Luckman J and Sorenson KC: Medical-surgical nursing, ed 3, Philadelphia, 1987, WB Saunders Co.
16. Lye M: Electrolyte disorders in the elderly, Clin Endocrinol Metab 13(2):377, 1984.
17. Martof M: Fluid balance, part 1, J Nephrol Nurs 2(1):10, 1985.
18. Maxwell MH and Kleeman CR: Clinical disorders of fluid and electrolyte metabolism, ed 4, New York, 1987, McGraw-Hill Inc.
19. Meites S: Pediatric clinical chemistry, Washington, DC, 1981, The American Association for Clinical Chemistry.
20. Mountcastle VB: Medical physiology, ed 14, St. Louis, 1980, The CV Mosby Co.
21. Murray RB, Huelskoetter MMW, and O'Driscol DL: The nursing process in later maturity, New Jersey, 1980, Prentice-Hall, Inc.
22. Olds SB et al: Maternal-Newborn nursing, ed 2, San Fransisco, 1984, Addison-Wesley Publishing Co Inc.
23. Perry AG and Potter PA: Clinical nursing skills and techniques, ed 2, St. Louis, 1990, Mosby – Year Book.
24. Phillips PA et al: Reduced thirst after water deprivation in healthy elderly men, N Engl J Med 311(2):753, 1984.

25. Phipps WJ, Long BC, and Woods NF: Medical-surgical nursing: concepts and clinical practice, ed 4, St. Louis, 1991, Mosby–Year Book.

26. Plumer AL and Cosentino F: Principles and practice of intravenous therapy, ed 4, Boston, 1987, Little, Brown & Co Inc.

27. Porth C: Pathophysiology: concepts of altered health states, ed 2, Philadelphia, 1986, JB Lippincott Co.

28. Ramsey JM: Basic pathophysiology, Palo Alto, Calif., 1982, Addison-Wesley Publishing Co Inc.

29. Rose BD: Clinical physiology of acid-base and electrolyte disorders, ed 2, New York, 1984, McGraw-Hill Inc.

30. Shapiro BA, Harrison RA, and Walton JR: Clinical application of blood gases, ed 3, Chicago, 1982, Year Book Medical Publishers Inc.

31. Sodeman WA, Jr. and Sodeman WA: Pathologic physiology: mechanisms of disease, ed 7, Philadelphia, 1985, WB Saunders Co.

32. Tilkian SM, Conover MB, and Tilkian AG: Clinical implications of laboratory tests, ed 4, St. Louis, 1987, The CV Mosby Co.

33. Underhill SL et al: Cardiac nursing, Philadelphia, 1982, JB Lippincott Co.

34. Whaley LF and Wong DL: Nursing care of infants and children, ed 4, St. Louis, 1991, Mosby–Year Book.

35. Widmann FW: Clinical interpretation of laboratory tests, ed 9, Philadelphia, 1983, FA Davis Co.

36. Wyngaarden JB and Smith LH: Cecil textbook of medicine, ed 18, Philadelphia, 1988, WB Saunders Co.

Index

Anterior fontanel, palpating of infant's, 89
Antidiuretic hormone, 36, 38, 39
    in fluid volume deficit, 83
    in fluid volume excess, 86, 105, 106
    in fluid volume imbalance, 82
    and urine, 36
Aramine; see Metaraminol, 124
Arterial oxygen tension, (Po$_2$) cf 66
Ascites, third spacing and, 112
Atom, 6
Atropine, dry mouth and, 36

B

Babinski's reflex, 155
Babinski's sign and hypomagnesemia,
    154-155
Base, 44
    proton acceptance, 45
Base bicarbonate, symbol for, 62
Bicarbonate, 55
Bicarbonate ions, 53
Blood gas analysis, 66-67
Body fluids
    constituents of, 6-12
    distribution of, 4-5
    loss of, 29-30
    movement of, 14-28
    sources of, 52
Body fluid amounts, total, 1
Body fluid compartments, 2-4, 12
Body water, total, 5
Bowel resection as cause of
    hypomagnesemia, 153
Bradycardia in hypomagnesemia, 156
Buffer system, 48, 49-51, 54, 55, 56
    major systems of, 50-51
    mechanism of action, 50-51

C

Calcitonin, 168
Calcium
    bound, 166
    functions of, 107
    as magnesium antagonist, 164
    recommended dietary allowance for, 173
    serum, sources of, 168;
        see also Serum calcium
Calcium bicarbonate, 49
Calcium deficit, 170-176;
        see also Hypocalcemia

Calcium excess (hypercalcemia), 176-182
Calcium gluconate, 174
    use of, in treating hyperkalemia, 146
Calcium imbalance, 165-183
    and bound calcium, 166, 167
    calcium deficit, 170-176
    hypercalcemia, 176-182; see also
        Calcium excess
Calcium stones, with hypercalcemia, 181
Cancer
    as cause of hypercalcemia, 177
    treatment of hypercalcemia in, 181
Capillary
    arterial end, hydrostatic and osmotic
        pressure in, 24
    hydrostatic pressure in arterial end, 24
    venous end, hydrostatic and osmotic
        pressure in, 25
Carbon dioxide
    buffer system and, 50
    normal content, 67
    in respiratory alkalosis, 59
Carbon dioxide tension (Pco$_2$), 66
Carbonate, buffer system and, 50
Carbonic acid(s) (H$_2$CO$_3$), 44, 49
    in respiratory acidosis, 57
    symbol for, 62
Carpal spasm, 172
Cathode, 8
Cations, 7, 9, 12
Cation-exchange resins, use of, in treating
        hyperkalemia, 146
Cell membranes, permeability, calcium
        and, 167
Cell nutrition, edema, effects of, 128
Cerebral function, disturbed, in fluid
        volume excess, 108
Chemical activity of electrolytes,
        measurement of; see Combining
        power of electrolytes
Chemical combining power, 12; see also
        Combining power of electrolytes
Chemical reactions, 2
Children, maintenance fluids in,
        calculation of, 29
Chloride (Cl), 8, 9, 14
Chvostek's sign
    hypomagnesemia and, 154-155
    in neuromuscular excitability, 172
Cl; see Chloride

Hemoglobin system, 51; *see also* Buffer
systems
Hemoglobin level, fluid volume, excess
and, 109
Homeostasis, 35-36
of body fluid volume, 36
Hormone(s)
adrenal cortical steroid, and potassium
excretion, 137
antidiuretic, and fluid volume
regulation, 36, 37
parathyroid
magnesium and, 150
and serum calcium, 169
Hydrochloric acid (HCl), 50
Hydrogen, 10
Hydrogen ion concentration; *see* pH
changes in, effects of, 46, 47
maintenance of, normal mechanisms
for, 48, 54
Hydrostatic pressure, 22, 24, 27, 34
Hyperalimentation
and hypocalcemia, 174
and hypomagnesemia, 152
Hypercalcemia
calcium stones in, 181-182
cardiac effects of, 179
causes of, 176-178, 183
factors leading to, 178
gastrointestinal effects of, 79
signs and symptoms of, 178-180, 182
treatment of, 180-182
Hyperkalemia
cardiac signs of, 147
causes of, 143-144
ECG changes in, 145
laboratory findings in, 145
treatment of, 145, 146
Hypermagnesemia, 162-165; *see also*
Magnesium excess
interventions for, 164
causes of, 162-163
and renal failure, 162
signs and symptoms of, 163-164
Hypernatremia, 126-129; *see also* Sodium
excess conditions related to, 126
symptoms of, 127
treatment of, 128-129
Hyperparathyroidism, primary, and
hypercalcemia, 177

Hyperpotassemia, 143 *see also*
Hyperkalemia; Potassium excess
Hypertonic solution, 19, 26
Hypocalcemia, 170-176; *see also* Calcium
deficit
causes of, 171
signs and symptoms of, 171-173, 175
treatment of, 174-175
Hypokalemia, 134-141; *see also* Potassium
deficit: Hypopotassemia
cardiac signs of, 138-139
causes for, 136
clinical signs and symptoms, 141-142
gastrointestinal signs of, 138
excretion, increased urinary, 137
respiratory signs of, 138
Hypomagnesemia, 151-161
cardiovascular signs of, 156
causes of, 152-154
signs and symptoms of, 154-156,
161
treatment of, 156-157
Hyponatremia, 120-126; *see also* Sodium
deficit
gastrointestinal symptoms of, 121
laboratory findings, 123
mild, symptoms of, 123
and orthostatic hypotension, 122
treatment of, 123-124
Hypopotassemia, 134; *see also* Potassium
deficit; Hypokalemia
Hypotension, as sign of
hypermagnesemia, 165
Hypothalamus
in fluid volume deficit, 85
and initiating thirst, 35
Hypotonic dehydration, 87
Hypotonic solution, 18, 26
Hypovolemia during third spacing, 113
Hypoxia in respiratory acidosis, 79
Hypertonic dehydration, 87

I

Imbalance, fluid and electrolytes, 32-34,
39-42; *see also* Fluid and electrolyte
imbalance
Immobilization, prolonged, as cause of
hypercalcemia, 178
Infants, fluid volume deficit in, signs of,
92

R

Rate of flow of intravenous fluids
  adjusting, 100-104
  calculating, 98-100
  mechanical factors affecting, 100
Renal calculi (kidney stones) in
      hypercalcemia, 179, 181-182
Renal disease as cause of hyponatremia,
      120
Renal failure as cause of
      hypermagnesemia, 162, 165
Renal insufficiency as cause of
      hypocalcemia, 171
Renal system, 49, 54, 55-56
  as defense mechanism in acid-base
      imbalance, 52-56
  of elderly person, 54
Renin, 119
Resorption
  nursing observations during, 114
  as second phase of third spacing, 113
Respirations, assessment of in acid-base
      imbalance, 74
Respiratory acidosis, 56-58, 63
  case study in, 79
  extracellular fluid, pH imbalance in, 57
  nursing care for, 68-70
  signs of, 68
Respiratory alkalosis, 58-60, 63
  case study in, 80
  extracellular fluid, pH imbalance in, 59
  nursing care for, 70-71
  signs of, 70
Respiratory depression in
      hypermagnesemia, 163
Respiratory failure during intravenous
      magnesium infusion, 160
Respiratory system, 48, 54, 55, 56
  as defense mechanism, 51-52

S

Saline
  isotonic, 18
  normal, 18
Semipermeable membranes, 3
Serum calcium
  concentration, factors controlling, 168
  sources of, 168
Serum calcium level, 166
Serum potassium level, normal, 139

Skin turgor as sign of sodium deficit, 122
Sodium (Na), 8, 9, 12
  aldosterone and, 37
  in fluids, isolation of, 120
  importance of, 124
  loss of, mechanisms for, 120
  regulation of, and fluid volume
      regulation, 119-120
Sodium bicarbonate ($NaHCO_3$), 49
  in metabolic acidosis, 60
Sodium chloride (NaCl), 6, 8, 9, 118
Sodium deficit, 120-126; *see also*
      Hyponatremia
  case study, 125
  laboratory findings in, 123
  signs and symptoms of, 121-123
  treatment of, 123-124
Sodium excess, 126-129; *see also*
      Hypernatremia
  treatment of, 128-129
Sodium imbalance
  case study, 130-131
  sodium deficit, 120-126
Sodium level, control of, 118
Solute, 14
Solution
  hypotonic, 18
  hypertonic, 19
  isotonic, 17-18
Solvent, 15, 16
Specific gravity, 20-21
Specific gravity of urine, normal, 84
Spironolactone, 129
Standard plasma bicarbonate (HCO_3), 66
  normal value, 67
Surgery, major, as cause of
      hypomagnesemia, 153

T

Tachycardia in hyponatremia, 122
Testosterone, use of, in treating
      hyperkalemia, 146
Tetany, 46
  in hypocalcemia, 171
Thiazides, 136
Third spacing, 112-114
  case study of, 116
  factors allowing, 112
  first phase, fluid volume shift during,
      112-113

Third spacing—cont'd
  hypovolemia during, 113
  resorption as second phase of, 113
  urine output during, 113
Thirst, 35-36
  atropine for, 36
  and extracellular fluid volume, 35-36
  fluid volume deficit and, 83, 85
  and hypothalamus, 35
Thyrocalcitonin; see Calcitonin
Total body water, 5
Total parenteral nutrition, hypocalcemia
      and, 174
Trauma as cause of hyperkalemia,
      143-147
Triamterene, 136
Trousseau's sign in hypocalcemia, 172
Tumors, effects of, on calcium release,
      177

U

Ulcerative colitis and potassium deficit, 41
Unconsciousness in acid-base imbalance,
      74
Urea, 6
Uremic acidosis, 60
Urine
  amount excreted in 24 hours, 31
  and magnesium excretion, 151
  output, normal, 31
  specific gravity of, normal, 84
  volume, regulation of, 36

Urine output
  during third spacing, 113
  pediatric, 93

V

Ventricular fibrillation, respiratory acidosis
      and, 68
Vitamin D
  calcium regulation and, 168-170
  deficiency of, hypocalcemia in, 170
  sources of, 169

W

Waste products, transportation of, 2
Water
  average amount taken in daily, 31
  distilled, 18-19
  and electrolytes, entering and leaving
      body, normal mechanism for, 28-32
  oral liquids, 28
  sources for, 28
Water and electrolytes, entering and
      leaving body, normal mechanism
      for, 28-32
Water deficit, severe, signs of, 86
Water in foods, 28
Water excess in fluid volume excess, 107
Water-excess syndrome, 109
Water intoxication, case study of, 115-116
Wrinkled skin as sign of dehydration in
      elderly, 90